Seven Days
of
Hospice

Seven Days of Hospice

A MEMOIR

D. M. Wilmes

Author of *Gone But Not Forgotten: A Christmas Story*

iUniverse, Inc.
New York Lincoln Shanghai

Seven Days of Hospice
A MEMOIR

iUniverse books may be ordered through booksellers or by contacting:

iUniverse
2021 Pine Lake Road, Suite 100
Lincoln, NE 68512
www.iuniverse.com
1-800-Authors (1-800-288-4677)

Because of the dynamic nature of the Internet, any Web addresses or links contained in this book may have changed since publication and may no longer be valid.

The views expressed in this work are solely those of the author and do not necessarily reflect the views of the publisher, and the publisher hereby disclaims any responsibility for them.

ISBN: 978-0-595-46373-2 (pbk)
ISBN: 978-0-595-70150-6 (cloth)
ISBN: 978-0-595-90666-6 (ebk)

Printed in the United States of America

To my mother,
Alice Elaine Wilmes.
We all miss you very much.

"Hope is not the conviction that something will turn out well, but the certainty that something makes sense regardless of how it turns out."

—*Vaclav Havel*

Introduction

My mother was an energetic woman, with verve beyond her years, who took great care of her health. For her, mammograms and physicals were as obligatory as Sunday Mass. They were faithfully scheduled, and she never missed any of them. Mom also had to have her kidneys checked each year to ensure the damage from childbirth had not worsened over time. The procedure was invasive, and she dreaded the annual visit, but she always received a clean bill of health.

Despite the toll her body and soul had endured delivering and rearing three boys and three girls, she was the most physically and mentally active grandmother anyone could ask for. With frequent doses of reading and aerobics, she exercised her mind and body. Armed with good health, new titanium knees, and laser-corrected eyes, Mom was ready to engage the autumn of her life with the energy of a teenager.

During one of her regularly scheduled routine examinations, the doctor discovered a small lump in her left breast. It was presumed to be another cyst. Mom had had a couple of them removed before, and this one seemed no more or less threatening than the rest. Cysts and other menacing but harmless physical nuisances were no big deal for a mother of six.

Outpatient surgery was scheduled to extract a sample of the foreign matter. As is standard medical practice, the tissue would be sent for analysis to determine whether it was cancer or not. Just the mention of the harmless word *cyst*, especially from those in the medical community, provides such a false sense of security. Like an umbrella, it's easy to hide under, protected from the ominous rain of disease affecting others.

How affirming it is to hear from our doctor, "It's probably just a cyst." It is equally reassuring to hear the same from supportive friends and family. What we often neglect, whether purposeful or not, is the stream of seemingly empty words that follow: "It's probably just a cyst, but we'll want to do a biopsy just in case." We were no different. Mom would go for a simple biopsy as she normally did, unaccompanied so as not to unnecessarily disturb any of her children or her husband from their important daily routines, confident that the tedious ordeal would be behind her in a day or so.

It was this visit that set off a rollercoaster of emotions, from extreme optimism to extreme hopelessness, our family had never before experienced. The outcome of the biopsy brought the worst possible news. As a result of that test, my mother, Elaine, was diagnosed with breast cancer in the spring of 2003.

A discouraging buzz spread quickly throughout our large family, and it left a perceptible trail of numbness along the way. The eight of us had been gifted with good health all of our lives, so it made the news difficult to digest. Something like this just wasn't supposed to happen to our family. It wasn't part of the script. In my version of our parents' chronicle, and I think for my siblings' as well, Mom and Dad were supposed to grow old together, just as our grandparents and great grandparents had done. Sure, there would be setbacks along the way, but cancer would not be found in the story line.

Surgery was immediately scheduled to determine the extent of her cancer. My mother's doctor and surgeons hoped that the cancer would be contained solely within the small lump, which would be completely removed. During the operation, surgeons would also check to see if cancer had already begun its destructive journey to other parts of her body. The lymph nodes, as described by the physicians, would provide clues about the extent to which the cancer had spread. Lymph nodes are the filters that collect and destroy bacteria and viruses and are an important line of defense when the body is fighting an infection, including a tumor. If the lymph nodes were healthy, chances were good that the cancer was self-contained.

It was a Monday morning when my father escorted Mom to the hospital for her surgery. It would be afternoon before we knew anything of certainty, and Mom didn't want her brood stirring about the waiting room, so all of us kids (the term reflects adolescent youth when in fact, we're all grown and most of us are married with children) reluctantly went to work. Dad promised he would call as soon as he knew something.

All morning I thought about Mom and the outcome of her surgery. She had lost several family members to cancer, including a brother she was very close to. Cancer and other foreboding diseases loomed over her side of the family and abruptly ended the young lives of those it captured. My dad's family, on the other hand, did everything that opposed a healthy lifestyle and lived long lives. A hearty dose of whole milk with coffee, eggs, sausage, bacon, lard, and cigarettes apparently discouraged cancer from entering their lives. I had always prayed that I was endowed with his genes.

I had just returned to my office from lunch when Dad called. He was very upset. He fought back as best he could, but a river of emotion was drowning him. In a wavering and dispirited voice, Dad managed to tell me the news.

Cancer was found in Mom's breast. Most of the lymph nodes under her arms appeared to be cancerous as well, including the important sentinel nodes. The surgeons forged ahead to remove them along with her breast. I left work immediately to be with him. My first thought, stemming from complete naivete, was that this was good news. After all, the doctors found more cancer and removed it. The more they removed, the better, I thought, even if it meant losing a breast.

A good friend and colleague of mine had been diagnosed with breast cancer several years ago. Listening to her, you knew she lived two lives—pre-cancer and post-cancer—and she wasn't afraid to share even the most intimate details of either. Prior to cancer she was a shy emotional wreck who folded and cried under the slightest banter. It would be safe to say she was a doormat—a victim of her own self-inflicted sensitivity. A young woman in her thirties, she underwent a mastectomy and months of chemotherapy. When all was said and done, she was cancer free.

Looking at her now, you would never know she had undergone anything of a significant medical nature beyond childbirth. Her personality took a complete about-face. Today she is a confident, outspoken, take-charge woman with energy beyond comprehension. She quit her job of over twenty years in quality control and testing to be an instructor to *Fortune 500* companies, covering topics in software development and best practices. She travels the country exposing all she meets with not only her knowledge but also her addictive exuberance and zest for life.

The way I figured it, Mom would undergo chemotherapy to prevent any further spread of cancer and, like my friend, would be renewed in the end. My friend was the only breast cancer survivor I knew personally. To me, her experience was the norm. I saw countless news reports and articles that validated it as well. A sea of breast cancer survivors gathered each year at the Susan G. Komen Race for the Cure in St. Louis, all wearing their familiar pink and white T-shirts. While some were still crusading the epidemic disease, most were survivors. Regardless of the medium or event, the stories seemed to depict the same theme—survival.

It wasn't until further discussions with my father in the waiting room, and the periodic visits from masked surgeons to update us on their progress, that I learned the seriousness of the cancer's progression and about the long, arduous journey to recovery Mom would endure.

Cancer had found its way to my mother as it had to members of her family and countless others. Yet I had always thought that Mom would escape the clutches of cancer. She had kept her mind and body healthy by exercising them both nearly every day. If she wasn't at aerobics class, on the treadmill, cleaning the house, or shopping, all executed with equal vigor, she was reading books. In fact, she read so many books that my father built her a library wall in their finished basement, which housed only a small portion of Mom's volumes of mystery, murder, and suspense. We often joked that Mom read enough Alfred Hitchcock that she could kill any one of us and get away with it scot-free. Being a devout Catholic all of her life eased any sense of suspicion.

In the past several years my mother had had both knees replaced (we called her "the bionic woman") and went through the long, painful process of physical therapy to use the new titanium hinges. She underwent Lasik surgery to bring her natural eyesight back to 20/20. She purchased a new luxury Mercury, began reengaging with her surviving sisters by going on mini-adventures together, applied for and received a passport, and, with Dad by her side, discovered the fun and camaraderie that could only be experienced on cruise ships.

After raising six children, she was finally reaping the rewards of frivolity life had to offer but was for so long postponed until we had all safely left the nest. Not your typical grandmother, she was the youngest sixty-five-year-old I had ever known.

The news spread quickly from cell phone to cell phone, and soon all of my brothers and sisters were milling about the hallways and waiting room. The surgery went on for hours. Each visit from the surgeons brought worse news—more evidence of cancer, more confiscation of tissue, and more tests. It wasn't until the final visit later that afternoon that brought a ray of hope to all of us. The surgeons, despite the mastectomy and evidence of cancer in the lymph nodes, did not see any more beyond the lymph nodes. Her organs appeared to be fine. If that was the case, her survival greatly improved, provided any remaining cancer could be eliminated. But it was imperative that cancer treatment start immediately.

As expected, test results on the removed breast tissue and lymph nodes proved the cancer was malignant, and so Mom's journey to recovery began. Once the treatment plan was established with her oncologist, a procedure was scheduled to insert a small plastic tube into a vein just below her neck. This would be the port where the chemotherapy substance would be injected. The port would eliminate the discomfort of having her veins stuck by needles each time the chemotherapy treatment was performed. It also provided an avenue for the medication to go directly into the blood supply entering the heart. From there, it could be distributed quickly and efficiently to the rest of the body.

Because of the type of cancer found in her breast, Mom was a prime candidate for a recently FDA-approved drug called Herceptin. It was a new type of therapy for women whose tumors had an abundance of HER2 protein. The drug, combined with chemotherapy, had shown signs of reducing the size of tumors, preventing cancer growth for a longer period of time, and helping women live longer than those who received chemotherapy alone. Mom's doctor backed an application to include my mother as part of a clinical study. Her application was approved. Mom would be getting the latest treatments available. It was a shot of hopeful optimism that we all needed.

For the next year, Mom received chemotherapy from a local cancer treatment center. On one occasion early in the therapy, when she still possessed a healthy physique and a full head of hair, I drove her to the center. The waiting room was completely full. Those of us accompanying patients stood against the wall beside our loved ones so we wouldn't take a chair away from those physically weakened by treatments.

A quick survey of the room disclosed pain and suffering I had never witnessed before—bald heads, draped skin, shrunken limbs, and lifeless eyes. Some of the women adorned their delicate heads with brightly colored wraps. It did little to brighten the room or to camouflage their condition. With so much physical deterioration, it was hard to estimate their ages.

One woman, one of few donning a flowering wrap to hide her hairless head, was paging through a fashion magazine. Her eyes and lips were made up as though she were prepared to go out on the town. At first glance, she appeared to be in her middle forties. A second look, one with a more analytical eye, suggested that she might have been in her twenties. It was difficult to picture her, or any of the others, in a state of perfect health. I wondered what they looked like before cancer. Considering the fatigued appearance of every patient in the room, I surmised that the effects of chemotherapy seemed to age the average person by at least ten years or more. I found it repulsive to think of Mom in that condition.

No one said a word to anyone else. They just stared straight ahead or scanned the waiting room magazines, anticipating their name to be called. I speculated as to why so many people who shared the common bond of cancer had nothing to share with one another. It wasn't your typical doctor's visit where the ailment of those around you was unknown. Everyone was there for the same thing. The only differences were the types of cancers and the ingredients in the vile concoctions injected to fight the disease.

Normally a watcher of others, a student of passersby, so to speak, I found it excruciating to peruse the patients in the room. My mother didn't belong here. This was a place for the sick and dying, not my mother. She didn't yet exhibit the physical attributes of a chemotherapy recipient. Had I not shepherded her into the room and stood beside her, one might have thought she was an escort herself. I wanted to grab her by the arm and lead her out of the dismal place.

Mom adored her doctors and the friendly nurses that she came to know from the frequent visits. I found it ironic that she could revere the people who made her so sick at times that she contemplated quitting the therapy sessions and letting nature take its course.

Despite Mom's revulsion to the treatments, though, she never gave up. For her, resignation wasn't an acceptable means for anything worthwhile. She was the sort who always saw a light at the end of each tunnel she confronted, but that didn't stop her from seeking affirmation. Perhaps it was a characteristic cultivated from living in the "Show Me" state for so long. She asked me frequent questions regarding my coworker who conquered the disease. I answered them the best I could. I had hoped that sharing my stories of her helped to provide an element of that light. It seemed everyone who had heard of Mom's plight had a story to share with her about a daughter, mother, cousin, in-law, aunt, or friend who had battled and beaten breast cancer.

Mom also made contact with other breast cancer survivors through the hospital outreach program, and she asked many questions of them. It was reaffirming to hear such positive outcomes. The stories were much the same. They all went through hell to get to healthy. The fact of the matter was, Mom and the rest of us were plotting a course through the unknown. If her story ended like all the others, the horizon looked promising. It was the voyage itself that scared us all.

She had her good days and her bad days, even though the good ones were greatly outnumbered. But the good days were very good, enabling her to get out of the house for a while and shop or visit with friends. She planned outings in advance, knowing almost to the hour when the nauseating effects of chemotherapy would begin and end.

She purchased two wigs when her hair loss began so that one would always be ready to go if the other needed styling. Although she never said it aloud to me, I could tell the wigs and prosthetic breast were embarrassing crutches. On those occasions where I stopped by the house unannounced, she would, in comedic fashion, adjust her wig and blouse when she answered the door.

As much as the good days were very good, the bad days were very bad. She could only lie in bed, or on the living room couch, and wait for the nausea to end. A few months before the discovery of cancer, Mom had purchased the new couch and recliner for the living room. She was proud of them, and rightfully so. They were firm, comfortable, well made, and grand replacements for the worn ones that had occupied the living room for so many years.

Several times, Mom cursed the new couch saying it would be the first thing to go after she healed. She had spent so much time on it ridding her system of the noxious chemicals that had been injected into her port, and watching hours of DVDs to pass the time, that she had come to loathe it.

By early summer, the last of the chemotherapy sessions was finally over and visits were reduced to Herceptin injections and follow-up visits to ensure her blood counts were not falling. After a few tests and a nod from her watchful oncologist, her battle was finally over. She was cancer free. Mom had joined the ranks of so many women who had engaged, and beaten, her foe.

Yet she despised the stripes she had earned. Some of us thought it would be appropriate to proudly display those looping pink ribbons that represent cancer survival. You see them everywhere—magnetically affixed to cars, pinned on collars and lapels, and printed on T-shirts. Mom wanted nothing to do with them. Perhaps they were painful reminders of a time she would just as soon forget. We never pressed the issue with her. We discreetly tucked away the pink ribbons and never mentioned them again.

Given a new life spiced with encouragement, Mom wasted no time making up for lost time. Her hair started to grow again, although sparse at best, and a life of normalcy as she had hoped began to slowly return. She, her closest sister, and several sisters-in-law founded a local chapter of the nationally prominent Red Hat Society—a fun-seeking society of women who gaudily dress in fanciful red hats from the Victorian era, purple dresses, and flare of the most extreme proportions. Together they donned their colorful garb and set out on road trips to do nothing less than celebrate life. They visited local wineries, restaurants, old town shops, and gambling boats. My mother became the "queen bee" of their chapter, a tribute given to the heir-apparent leader of the flock.

Mom and Dad set out on cruises to Alaska, Australia, and the Caribbean. They befriended couples that were either battling breast cancer or had survived it. E-mails were exchanged long after the cruises had reached their final shore to keep in touch and offer support to one another. Life was returning to normal, for Mom and for all of us. In fact, it is safe to say it was better than normal. We all had a better sense of life's fragility.

It wasn't long after she was given a clean bill of health that Mom started to feel weak again. She felt tired most of the time and just couldn't escape the grip of fatigue. The oncologists insisted it was residual from the chemotherapy. They convinced her to wait it out, as it would eventually pass. She fought it the best she could, but even her newly found appetite for life couldn't overcome the exhaustion.

Based on the symptoms Mom described, her physician thought it might be depression. He prescribed a mild antidepressant and asked her to check back in a few weeks. Being unfamiliar with the symptoms of depression, Mom trusted the diagnosis and took the medication. It didn't help. The weakness she felt never dissipated. The longer she waited, the more concerned she and Dad became.

By late August, the fatigue was getting the best of her, and she convinced her oncologist that something was definitely wrong. They ordered a series of tests, including a CT scan and an MRI, to see what was ailing her. Mom was extremely claustrophobic and dreaded the MRI more than any other test. It was all she could talk about. Whatever sedatives was normally used, Mom was going to insist they double the dose for her. I thought it was odd that after all she had endured to date, she dreaded the enclosed space inside the MRI the most.

The news was devastating. Scans confirmed bone cancer this time. We couldn't believe it. Chemotherapy had not driven

cancer from Mom's body as we had thought. Instead it bur-
rowed deeper into her system. It pierced our family in the heart
and completely deflated our recently acquired high spirits.

Another round of chemotherapy sessions was ordered to
combat her advancing disease. If anything positive came from
her new diagnosis, it was that her type of cancer was slow to
spread. Chemotherapy could slow the growth even more and
provide her years of quality life. There was evidence that people
with bone cancer lived many years with the disease. It was also
possible, although only remotely, for it to go into remission.
Although the doctors never indicated how long Mom had to
live, they suggested that it was possible she could grow old with
the disease. As reluctant as she was to start chemotherapy all
over again, she wasn't about to let her latest disease take anything more away from her.

Mom started the regimen again, only this time the effects
were extreme. Several times during the chemotherapy treatments her blood cell counts fell to dangerously low levels. At
one point, she was rushed to the hospital because she was barely
responsive. She fell terribly weak and her appetite was under-
standably diminished. It was the first time she had hinted that
death would be better than going through the misery and pain
of chemotherapy.

The treatments had gone on for so long, and the effects were
so lethal, she was ready to quit. Intravenous drips, blood trans-
fusions, and steroid therapies were used to combat the undesirable developments and helped get her past the episodes of
weakness and defenselessness. Mom had to force herself to eat

to prevent any relapses of the side effects. It was dreadful for her to swallow even her favorite foods. It seemed to us that the treatments were just too toxic. Chemotherapy, we thought, was killing her faster than the cancer.

After some dangerous moments and a myriad of treatment combinations, Mom's oncologist was finally able to stabilize her health to what it was when she was first on chemotherapy for breast cancer. She still went through periods of nausea, which was to be expected, but it wasn't anything like her recent bouts. In fact, a short time after her health had stabilized the oncologist suggested that chemotherapy treatments might be nearly complete. They hinted each time she went in that the next time could be her last.

Mom was encouraged by the news, but every time she went in thinking that the visit might be the final one, her doctor ordered one more. One more turned into one more, which turned into one more. It didn't take long for Mom to grow tired of the cycle of empty predictions and miscalculations.

She said several times in disgust, "I'll probably be on chemotherapy the rest of my life."

I'm sure it seemed that way to her. It seemed like a lifetime to me already. She kept as optimistic as she could, however, hoping that the ordeal would soon be behind her.

In early November, when a truly meaningful Thanksgiving and Christmas were just around the corner, life dealt us another one of its unwelcome surprises. Mom began to weaken even more. Her speech began to slur, although barely noticeable at first. Bottled water and soft drinks were always at arm's length. When the uncontrollable slurring crept into her conversation, she took a drink of whatever she had on hand and followed it with an offhanded claim that her mouth was dry. She unconvincingly asserted that the dryness was yet another effect of chemotherapy. None of us believed it, since she had never shown signs of slurring before. Dad was concerned that she might have had a mild stroke. Mom scoffed at the idea, insisting it was residual, and that it would eventually pass.

I remember thinking, "Now what? What more could this woman possibly bear?" Doctors were puzzled at the turn of events and issued a series of tests. To add to her fear, the tests would also reveal if more cancer was present.

"I will not go through chemo again," she insisted. "I don't care if they find more cancer, I simply won't do that again."

We tried to convince her that we were not going to give up so easily, that we wanted to have our mother around for a very long time. But I knew in my heart that if it were me, I would have reached the same conclusion.

I can only recall two instances when good news had ever come to our family since Mom was diagnosed with cancer. The first was the day she was determined to be cancer free. The second was the day the results of her tests showed that no new cancer was present. We were all so relieved. It was a shot of hope we all needed. Mom wouldn't have to go through another sequence of chemotherapy.

That glimmer of hope, however, was quickly overshadowed by the fact doctors still didn't know what was wrong with her.

While each one negated the possibility of cancer, they were also disappointingly inconclusive. The slow methodical nature of today's medical community, especially when transferring a patient from one medical discipline to another, only made us all the more anxious. Test intervals spanned several days and left a series of professionals stumped by her condition. Mom's health, and our frustration, worsened as time went on.

By this time, Thanksgiving was just two weeks away. Mom and Dad had planned on hosting the holiday at their house for all thirty-plus people, like they did every year since I could remember. It was a much anticipated family tradition, and, each year, Mom went all out for the event by setting out her best dinnerware and preparing nearly every culinary delight from scratch. It was evident by this time that she would not be able to cater such a large affair. Her health had deteriorated to the point that it was difficult for her to move around on her own.

Dad asked if we could hold it at our house. We gladly obliged. My wife, Patti, and I set out to rearrange our house to accommodate the large gathering. As Thanksgiving approached, I took days off work to help prepare the feast. Patti and I looked forward to having everyone over, and we wanted to make this Thanksgiving extra special for Mom and Dad.

We joined two long tables together to form one massive contiguous slab that stretched from the kitchen into our adjoining living room. We set out our best china dishes, silverware, and glassware. Chilled wine, pumpkin bread, cranberries, and customary condiments were placed at frequent intervals to limit the passing of food from one end of the room to the other. No detail was left unanswered. It was just as Mom would have done.

On the eve of Thanksgiving, Patti and I heated the large roasting ovens borrowed a week before from Dad. They were now brimming with pulled turkey and Mom's special raisin bread dressing that I had attempted to do her proud by duplicating.

As we readied the house for the holiday affair, the phone rang. It was Dad. He broke the news to us that they would probably not be able to make it. Mom had become considerably weaker, and Dad was deeply concerned because her slurring had worsened. He asked us to continue with the holiday feast for the rest of the family. If she was able, they would come, but the probability was low. I tried to query Dad for answers, but he kept his voice low and only answered with brief and awkward replies. Once I realized he was intentionally shielding his conversation, as well as his concern, from Mom, I grudgingly tapered my inquiry.

Mom had batlike senses. Perhaps it came from raising six children. It was difficult to sneak anything past her. In any case, Dad wasn't able to speak freely to me, and I understood. After we hung up, my heart sank. It wouldn't be the same without them. It angered me that the doctors could find nothing when it was apparent something was obviously wrong. It would be a melancholy Thanksgiving at best, and I wanted to cancel it. How could any of us celebrate the holiday without them? Per Dad's wishes, however, we reluctantly went on with our plans.

By early afternoon of Thanksgiving, family members began to arrive, all bearing homemade side dishes, desserts, and spirits. Soon, brothers, sisters, spouses, and children bustled about the house. Wine bottles were uncorked, while warming trays dispensed aromas of sweet potatoes and casseroles. The walls echoed the rumors of Mom's latest condition, and it was all we could talk about. It dampered the normally festive occasion and the tone was subdued. Mom and Dad were always the nucleus of any family get-together, and it seemed disrespectful to be celebrating the holiday without them.

Just when we thought all had arrived who would arrive, the doorbell rang. It was Dad at our doorstep. Mom was clutching his arm.

"You made it!" I exclaimed while opening the door.

Others heard the announcement and rushed to the entry way. What I saw next nearly brought tears to my eyes. Dad led his beloved wife into the corridor. She could barely walk on her own and shuffled across the tile floor.

"I made it," she said with a smile. Her words were so slurred, I could hardly understand her. It was as if she were drunk on holiday wine.

I hugged her and welcomed her. I could tell it pained her to return the gesture. Every movement was slow and labored. It was as though she had aged forty years since I'd seen her only a few days ago. She even made light of her speech.

"I must have started drinking without you," she joked.

I wanted to crawl into a hole and cry. Whatever was afflicting her had reduced her to a shell of an old woman who could barely walk, much less speak. We were all aghast, but we hid it the best we could with love and affection.

We tried to carry on as usual on that Thanksgiving Day, drinking wine, overindulging on pecan and pumpkin pie, telling stories of the past, laughing and joking, but Mom's condition weighed heavily on all of us. Dad, who had quit smoking years ago, had started again. Those of us who smoked, and even those who didn't, met with him on the deck each time he had a cigarette. He tried to keep his smoking from Mom, although she knew what he was doing and rarely said anything. He was so upset. Several times he cried. He was lost and, like us, wanted to know what was wrong.

At one point Dad gathered all of us children on the deck and explained that doctors would perform a brain scan the following day. Once again, they would be looking for cancer, although nerve damage was another possible culprit. As much as we tried to cling to the latter prognosis, Dad stressed several times that nerve damage was a very remote possibility. He negated it as though he had already been informed of the results from the pending test. Dad was astute at reading people and understanding what is conveyed between the lines. He must have picked up on something the doctor had said, as he never seriously considered the possibility nerve damage.

Later in the afternoon, Mom mentioned the same thing. Her outlook was always positive, and with a sense of humor.

"They're going to do a brain scan," she said. Apparently we didn't disguise our concerned expressions very well. "Oh, don't worry. I'm sure it's just nerve damage or something. I think they just want to see if there really is a brain up there."

She said she felt fine, other than just being tired all of the time and unable to speak clearly. To her, it didn't have the familiar signature of cancer.

Already aware of Dad's version, we supported her in her theory and never let on we were informed otherwise. That was one of the hardest things I've ever had to do. Mom knew they were looking for cancer, but I wasn't sure if she was protecting us or honestly held hope that it was something less destructive. Whatever her reasoning, the word *cancer* never escaped her lips.

By late afternoon, Mom was tiring and asked to go home. We wanted her to stay longer, but our persuasions were not enough to overcome her fatigue. Dad dutifully fetched Mom's coat from the hall closet, carefully lifted her from her chair, and wrapped it around her shoulders. She didn't have the strength to lift her arms into the sleeves. We bid our extended farewells, indulging in as many hugs as slices of pie we had eaten that day, as Dad escorted his frail wife out of our house and into the car. It was heart-wrenching to watch her leave in such a fragile condition. I prayed that tomorrow's tests would finally bring an answer.

The following day, results from the scan showed inflammation of the meninges. Doctors first thought that Mom had some form of meningitis. Whether viral or bacterial, it was a dangerous and life-threatening disease, even for healthy individuals. Given Mom's weakened condition and depleted immune system, they immediately scheduled a lumbar puncture, or spinal tap, to prove or disprove the theory. If it was what they speculated, it would be critical that Mom get intensive medical attention. As a precautionary measure, she was admitted to the hospital so that the medical staff could keep a close eye on her.

Mom was in the hospital awaiting the results of her lumbar puncture when I went to see her. Dad intercepted me at the door and escorted me down the hall away from Mom's private room. It was then he broke down. He put his hand on my shoulder and drew me in close. I could feel myself wanting to back away, but I didn't. I froze. The lumbar puncture provided the answer, and it was what we all feared it to be. Brain cancer. We held each other more tightly than ever before as Dad cried on my shoulders. He explained the best he could as he cried.

I was in complete shock. The news didn't register right away. I asked him how long she had to live. The question was purely involuntary. It just came out. It was as if someone else asked the question and forced it through my lips. Through the sorrowful sobbing of this horribly broken man, he replied it could be four months, or it could be four weeks. No one knew for certain.

For me, time stood eerily still. I stood erect, wrapped in my father's arms, and felt nothing. Swathed in complete emptiness, I felt that my soul, my heart, and my mind had been siphoned from me. I was nothing more than an empty cocoon. I searched for answers, questions, anything that would put some logic to this horrid news. Nothing came. Not even tears. After a few more minutes of embrace, we released our clutch on each other and gathered our senses.

"We need to be strong now," he stated as he soaked up his tears with his handkerchief. "She doesn't know everything, and the doctor doesn't want us to say anything until he knows for sure."

Dad went on to explain that the doctor was waiting for some additional test results to come back. As it turned out, the doctor had just left prior to my arrival. He had explained privately to Mom and Dad that cancer was found in her central nervous system and in the fluid surrounding her brain and spinal cord. It was this cancer that was impacting her speech and causing her fatigue. Despite the bad news, he wanted to wait on a few more test results before giving a firm diagnosis, which he would do first thing tomorrow.

The grimmest of news followed. There were no treatments for her type of cancer. After the meeting with both of them, the doctor had pulled Dad into the waiting room and confided that he gave her little chance of surviving. Chemotherapy treatments or injections couldn't fight the cancer because the brain and spinal cord were contained in their own protective shell. If it was what he believed it to be, Mom would have three to four months to live, but depending on the speed of the cancer's horrific consumption, possibly much less. It was crucial, though, per the doctor's stern suggestion, that he be the one to break the news to Mom.

Denial immediately consumed me. "How can he say that when he doesn't have all of the test results back?" I contended.

"Maybe chemotherapy can help keep it from spreading. At least for a while. Doesn't she deserve that chance?"

Dad smiled at my naivete through his red and moistened eyes. "He's seen this enough times to know. But he also said she would feel no pain. Thank God for that." His voice trembled. Grief and tears returned to his face. "Go in and talk to her. I need to freshen up before I go back in there." He rubbed my shoulder and started to weep. "Diane and Laura are in the cafeteria downstairs. They already know. I need to see how they are doing. Be strong, okay?"

Dad walked off to erase as much of the sadness from his face as he could and comfort my sisters who were also struggling with pain. I stood in the hall and watched as he disappeared around the corner. Then, I turned toward the entrance to Mom's darkened room. I didn't want to go in. What would I say? What could anyone say that could make this any more bearable? No one should have to face a loved one knowing their life is near its end while they cling desperately to an empty vessel of hope.

Or did she know? With no conclusive results, did she feel that she still had a chance? No, she has to know! We're all accustomed to reading between the lines. When a doctor says it could be this or it could be that, common sense always seems to step in and formulate a logical path for us. She's not stupid. She heard what the doctor said. Like a derailed train, thought after thought smashed into the next, each one hurled into the air and landing into oblivion. It was as if I had no control over my own mind.

While I was standing in the center of the hallway contemplating my entrance, a nurse on her rounds quietly stepped around me. She gave me that smile I've grown to despise. It's the sympathetic smile—the one people offer when they know of your misfortune and choose not to say anything. It's the same meaningless smile that funeral directors give to surviving family members who have lost loved ones. I'd seen it so many times before as pall bearer to my grandparents, uncles, and aunts. I know they meant to be sympathetic, but I still despised it.

That's when it hit me. This was not some sadistic dream I would awaken from. It was real. My mother was going to die. She was lying alone in a hospital room while sand pooled to the bottom of her hourglass. I had no time to waste. I took a deep breath and walked in.

Mom managed to smile when I entered the room. I went to her side, bent across her bed, and held her tight.

"I'm so sorry. If I could take this away from you, I would, Mom." And I would have without so much as a blink. This was not a fair ending for someone who had spent most of her young life struggling and sacrificing to raise a large family. She had just begun to live, and I wanted desperately to give her life back to her.

She insisted it wasn't over yet. She held hope that additional chemotherapy might stop the growth of her new cancer and that she would be with us for many more years. It pained me to hear her say that. I wanted to believe it, but I couldn't. So many times, hope had dissipated into thin air. What appeared to be a harmless cyst turned out to be a tumor. What cancer was thought to be contained in one tiny lump had spread to the lymph nodes and beyond. When the cancer was finally destroyed, it returned, but with a vengeance. It just wasn't fair.

So many times I'd heard success stories, whether on television or in my own personal life, of women who beat breast cancer. They were everywhere. Despite the staggering number of women who contract breast cancer every year, nearly that of epidemic proportions, the success stories were so prevalent that it seemed death from breast cancer was nonexistent. I hadn't heard of any women dying from it. I had only heard of women surviving it. So why, then, wasn't my mother one of the survivors? What was so different about my mother, who had kept herself both mentally and physically fit, that she couldn't win the battle? Question after question raced through my mind, yet none of them was followed by answers. All the while, Mom continued to fight with optimistic determination.

"Oh, don't you worry. I'll beat this," she said with a weakened smile. Her eyes told a different story, though. They lacked the confidence she once had. She knew.

One by one her children trickled into the room. Dad had sequestered each one before they reached the door and broke the news to them. I could read it in their faces as they walked in. They had the same poorly camouflaged look of shock and despair as I'm sure I did. Despite the doctor's prophecy, however, conversations that night were kept upbeat. We all rallied around the possibility that the doctors would slow the effects of the newly found cancer and permit our mother to be with us for a while. As was Mom's nature, she kept the mood buoyant with encouraging words. Anything less was unacceptable. No one mentioned death that evening. We talked only of long life and happiness.

The news came as expected the following evening. I arrived just moments after the doctor had left. What little hope we caressed last night had been torn from our clutching arms. My three sisters and younger brother were at her bedside weeping. Dad was stroking Mom's head whispering, "I love you," repeatedly. They had heard the doctor's prognosis firsthand. As I approached the foot of her bed, Dad shared the revelation through a mountain of raw emotion and despair, all the while never turning away from her.

"There is nothing they can do. She's not going to be with us much longer." His head lowered to Mom's breast, and he bellowed a laden cry.

I bent over to hug Mom. All I could do was apologize and tell her I loved her as tears swelled within me. Encouragement from the previous evening, as remote as it might have been, was completely destroyed. The festering wound of Mom's imminent death revealed by Dad's visit in the hallway was reopened and now pulsated with a disturbing reality. Without knowing all of the facts, I joined my family in the crowded hospital room and began the painful acceptance of Mom's limited existence.

It was a quiet evening, and a meaningful one. We cried often. We exchanged feelings we had never said aloud before. We talked openly of her greatness as a mother. We reminded her of the legacy of children, and grandchildren, she had created. We each shared personal feelings we had never shared before. Mom listened and occasionally flashed a melancholy smile, but each one slowly transformed to an empty gaze into the nothingness in front of her. Her thoughts were elsewhere. She just stared straight away.

Every once in a while she massaged her temples and forehead as if in deep contemplation. I wondered what she was thinking and where her mind was going. I couldn't imagine being told my days were numbered. It just wasn't fair. We couldn't stop touching her. Each one of us held on to her and caressed her arms, legs, and face. I suppose we were all touching her for different reasons. I wanted to absorb the blackness from her body and drive it out. I prayed to God to let me trade places with her. I also wanted to hold her and feel her warmth. There is nothing in this world like a mother's tenderness.

Later that night Dad privately shared the outcome of the doctor's visit. Her life expectancy was estimated at two weeks to two months. That news alone stunned me. The four-month to four-week window from yesterday was cut in half. Without knowing it, we had already lost valuable time. We could do nothing more than to accept the fact that Mom was dying. It was a difficult reality to consume and repulsive in every sense.

A hospice administrator visited us the next morning to help us through the process of getting Mom home and taking care of her. I hated hearing the word mentioned in front of Mom. *Hospice* is such a passive word, but its meaning is so haunting. It is the preparation for one's death. We were making plans to prepare for Mom's death. It seemed wrong to talk about it openly in front of her, but I suppose it was necessary.

After some empathetic words, most of which breezed by me or slid off my new skin of resentful Teflon, the administrator went through her checklist of items we might need—a bedpan, walker, wheelchair, bedding options, and more. Each item was discussed in detail, almost too much detail, I thought, and was followed by some scribbled notations on her clipboard.

Do we really need a fifteen-minute discussion on a wheelchair, I thought to myself? If we used it, great. If we didn't, so be it. I wanted to move the conversation along as quickly as possible, if not for Mom's sake, then my own, although I don't think Mom heard much of it. She was still locked in her silent gaze, nodding only when we needed her approval. It seemed as if we were scraping open a lesion over and over with each item on the list.

With Dad and five of his children readied at the helm, Mom was privileged to have so many people who could take care of her. The administrator commented on it as well. We were lucky in that regard. But with six people came six different opinions and a myriad of memories. Conversations of hospice care often drifted off topic with each of us, including myself, sharing abstract thoughts and memories that almost always ended with tears. The hospice administrator quietly obliged our less-than-focused discussions and reeled us in when the reminiscence subsided.

She explained numerous times that they would provide no service, or apparatus, for prolonging Mom's life. "Our goal is to make her as comfortable as possible," the woman repeated over and over. I cringed every time she said it. Sometimes our questions inadvertently provoked that response.

"What about one of those intravenous poles on wheels?" I asked.

"You won't need one unless she is in pain and needs pain medication administered through a drip. Since your mother is in no pain, a pole won't be necessary. We want to make your mother as comfortable as possible ..."

We were slowly and painfully being deprogrammed. There would be no monitors, no intubation, no attempts to extend her life. Every heart-wrenching reminder, and there were many that morning, thrust the determined blade of realization deeper into my chest until my soul was nearly lifeless. Our mission was not to save Mom, but to comfort her, and release her, to the great beyond as quietly, painlessly, and lovingly as possible.

This is her story—the last seven days of my mother's life.

Saturday, December 3

I arrived at the hospital a few minutes after seven o'clock in the morning. Visiting hours didn't officially begin until eight, but, fortunately, this hospital was not a stickler for such rules. It was decided last night that I would stay with Mom to ensure that her release and transfer went off as planned. Once the nursing staff received the go-ahead call from the doctor, the ambulance service would be dispatched to bring her home. It was my responsibility to make sure that happened with as little delay as possible.

While I was at the hospital, Dad and my sisters prepared the house for Mom's arrival. The hospice company was to deliver the necessary hardware as determined by the family the day before—a motorized hospital bed with adjustable rails, an air mattress especially designed to minimize bed sores by oscillating pressure points to different parts of the body in a continuous but slow motion, a bedpan, a bedside mobile cart, and a walker. We wanted Mom to be as comfortable as possible, as was drilled into us by the hospice administrator, and it was agreed the living room would be large enough to accommodate the equipment and suit the need.

While Dad and my sisters were busy cleaning the house, moving furniture, and anticipating the arrival of equipment, I was to keep my mother company. Once again, I paused at the entrance to her room. Once again, I pondered the right things to say. Once again, they never came. In that moment of contemplation, it dawned on me that there are no right things to say, only things to say. Say them now, I thought, and say them frequently. You would think that would be obtrusively evident. Why would it be that I would waste precious time thinking about what to say? Perhaps it was the hope that her outcome might be different. Perhaps saying the right thing would, somehow, make her situation better. Whatever it was, it was a complete waste of time. I gathered my senses and walked in.

"Good morning, Mom. I'm here to bust you out."

"Good," she murmured, "I want to get out of here." She fashioned a hint of a smile as I rounded her bed.

I gave her a hug and told her I loved her. We held each other tightly. I didn't want to let her go. I could feel the warmth of her neck against my cheek, and I didn't want the moment to end. It was a tender embrace only a mother and child could know. An emotional rush came over me and my tears returned. I couldn't fight them back any longer.

"I love you," I whispered again in her ear.

She repeated the meaningful words to me and held me tighter. When I think of Mom today, I go back to that precious moment. For a time of so much hopelessness and despair, it felt so warm and perfect.

We talked for thirty minutes or so. It could have been longer, I don't recall. It was one of those rare occasions when time pressured neither of us. The only engagement of any importance was getting her home, and even that was out of our hands. I had called my manager the day we learned of Mom's ill-fated future. He had granted me as much time as I needed to be with my family. I am one who, even on vacation, keeps track of business correspondence on a daily basis. Checking voice mail and e-mail were common practices for me on days off. Not this time. When I had left the office the previous Thursday, I left it all behind. I thought of nothing but Mom and Dad. It was as if I didn't have a job to worry about, and it was the first time since I can remember actually putting my job responsibilities on hold. It permitted me the gift of total concentration on Mom and her needs, and I appreciated the freedom immensely.

In the brief pauses in our conversation, I asked her if she needed anything. I must have asked her a hundred times, if not a thousand, "Can I get you anything?" "Do you need anything?" "Is there anything I can do for you?" I caught myself at one point and thought she might be growing tired of my repeated inquiries, but I could tell by the way she answered, she wasn't annoyed at all.

It was also during those silent moments that I surveyed my mother. I couldn't help but notice the physical changes that had taken place over the past few months. Pale, translucent skin was a stark contrast where soft auburn hair, and thick lashes, once blossomed. Her cheeks, once plump and blush, and youthfully pillaring a beautiful white smile, were now descended and sunken, forcing an uncontrollable grimace. Her large pearl-bejeweled brown eyes conveyed the heavy fatigue cancer had befallen on her. Numerous bruises from the poking and prodding of needles speckled her arms. It's disturbing enough to see how corrosive cancer can be to those it victimizes. It was exponentially more disturbing to see cancer consume my mother, and I didn't want to see her that way. If a friend of Mom's had happened upon her at this moment, they probably wouldn't have recognized her.

I left the room for a moment to check on the status of her departure. The nurse indicated that the doctor had not yet called, so she offered to call the doctor herself. She promised to keep me informed when she knew something and went right to work. I returned to Mom's room and updated her on the progress. I could tell she was troubled by the delay. She repeated several times that she just wanted to go home, and I wanted badly to make that happen for her.

Just a few minutes later, the nurse entered the room with a proud grin. As it happened, she was able to locate the doctor and received approval to dismiss Mom from the hospital.

"I'll get the discharge papers ready for you to sign. After that, we'll call the ambulance for your transfer. How does that sound?" The nurse seemed to be as pleased as we were with the speedy progression of events. She knew Mom was ready to go home and I appreciated her efforts.

It was the news Mom and I had hoped to hear. I immediately called Dad to let him know what had transpired. The hospice company was already on site, setting up the bed as we talked.

Dad was glad to hear that everything was falling into place. He repeated our conversation to my sisters. I could sense an air of excitement for all of us. Mom was coming home.

The nurse returned with a mound of paperwork related to the discharge. She handed Mom the clipboard and tethered pen, and asked her to sign on all areas marked with an X. Mom tried her best to sign the topmost piece of paper but could only manage an illegible scribble. It looked like that of small child who had no knowledge of penmanship or the alphabet.

"I can't even sign my own name," she sighed in disgust. Mom let the clipboard fall to her lap.

I asked the nurse if it was acceptable for me to sign the papers for Mom. With an understanding nod, she gathered the forms from Mom's lap and handed them to me. I glanced at Mom while flipping through the paperwork. She stared at the wall opposite me. I could see the disappointment in her eyes. I began endorsing the documents as quickly as possible to try and put the awkward moment behind us. It pained me to see her stare into the void. Although her face was expressionless, her eyes shifted about as though she were searching for something.

She had had an artistically caressed calligraphic style of handwriting. Her signatures had been masterfully crafted with looping strokes of style and grace. Mom religiously sent birthday cards to her children and grandchildren. I always recognized her inscription immediately. I didn't need to look at the return address to know the source of the letter, and the accurate timing of delivery revealed its content. I hadn't known until that moment that her ability to write had deteriorated as quickly as her speech. It was yet another confirmation that Mom's journey to death had already begun its relentless march.

I handed the clipboard and pen to the nurse. With signed discharge papers in hand, she scurried off to dispatch the ambulance and closed the door behind her.

"You'll be home soon," I reassured Mom while stroking her arm. She never broke from her fixation on the wall. My heart sank to the pit of my stomach and numbness seized me. I sat next to her and caressed her without saying a word. Her mind was in a place I couldn't fathom being. Nothing I could say was going to bring her out of it. I hoped that, by touching her, I was communicating what I felt.

The discomforting silence was interrupted when the nurse returned. Her news was unfavorable. The ambulance was transferring a patient to another hospital fifteen miles away. Depending on the nature of the call, it could be some time before they would be able to shuttle Mom. If they were not called away on another emergency, Mom's transportation home would be next. I remembered passing through the first floor emergency waiting room on my way to Mom that morning. For an early sunny Saturday morning, the ward was already half occupied by the sick and injured who were waiting to receive remedial attention. I prayed for a lull in emergency medical care, just long enough to get my mother home.

Mom and I were once again alone in her darkened room. For a few moments we had nothing to say. I held her hand and stroked her arm, recently bruised from the intravenous lines that had been removed earlier that morning. Without any warning or perceptible trigger, a sudden rush of emotion came over me. It was deafening, but void of sound. It was dizzying, but with nothing to see. It filled the room and spilled out into the hallway, but there was nothing to touch. I had never felt anything like it.

Mom and I were completely alone, and it was then I chose to empty my soul to her. I began to tell her that I was the person I was because of her. I told her that all of her children were successful, happy, and healthy human beings because of her devotion as a mother. I told her repeatedly that I loved her. The more I talked, the more I began to well up. My eyes pooled with tears, and my heart raced. I had never opened up to her like that before. Shamefully, these were new and foreign words. Perhaps that is why it seemed so painful. I should have done this before, and with frequency, but the time had never come. The opportunity had never presented itself. It hurt that I waited until now to tell her these things. It wasn't that we never shared close moments of tenderness and warmth, but they were never as intimate as this moment. They were never as brazenly honest and open.

Our family convened every holiday—Christmas, Thanksgiving, some Labor Days and Fourth of Julys, Easter, Father's Day, and Mother's Day. Except for my youngest sister and her husband who lived in the adjacent county, we all lived within the same city limits. It wasn't as though family members were strewn about the country. We gave gifts, told stories, sipped wine, and shared wonderful moments together. But to really sit down, one on one, and share our most intimate feelings was rare if nonexistent, at least for me. I was never the sort to express myself that way, until now. That is what I regretted most. With each confession of love and affection, my mother smiled and told me she understood. The fact was, I had never said these things before. They were, for the most part, assumed. But now, she knew. Now, we were both hearing it firsthand. It was the tenderest moment I had ever shared with her. It was truly a spiritual union of souls.

There came an echoed knock at the door. The interruption was like that of a gentle tug attempting to lead me away from a vivid dream. It was distracting, and I chose to ignore it. The knuckled thump against the solid wood door returned, this time more firm and prevalent. I stopped at the passageway of consciousness and paused to look one more time at a world I might never see again. It was a world of pure honesty, intimacy, and resolution. It was a moment filled with silent declarations of enduring love and affection. My mother and I connected in a way we had never done before. The door to her room swung slowly open. A faint light started to fill the room. I knew which direction to go, but it was with great reluctance. I didn't want the experience to end and hoped we would have another soon.

I turned toward the opened door. It was the nurse. She announced that the ambulance had arrived and that we needed to prepare for Mom's transfer. It was untimely news, but welcomed. Before we had a chance to dry our eyes, a uniformed man and woman appeared at the doorway with a mobile stainless steel bed between them. They were the paramedics we were waiting for, and they instantly lit up the dull beige room with bright smiles and humorous retorts about each other. They were like Will and Grace. They constantly ribbed one another and tried to see which one could outwit the other.

"We would have been here sooner but," the male paramedic motioned with his thumb to his female partner, "you know how women drivers are."

"Don't say that! She won't want to ride with us. Really, I am a good driver. I just have a lousy navigator."

Mom enjoyed the friendly banter and even threw in a few jabs of her own. I stepped out of the room while they lifted her from her hospital bed to the ambulance gurney. While waiting in the hallway, I called Dad to let him know Mom was on her way. The news brought him relief. His wife was finally coming home. During our conversation, I could hear laughter coming from Mom's room. The nurse, the paramedics, and my mother were having a good time. It sounded more like a party than anything else, and it made me laugh.

"What's going on?" Dad asked.

"I'm not sure, but Mom and the paramedics are having a good time in there."

"That sounds like Mom," Dad laughed. "Okay, I'll see you back here at the house."

Soon after, Mom was wheeled out of the room and still carrying on with entertaining paramedics. They paused in front of me so I could kiss her good-bye.

"I'll see you at home, Mom. I love you."

I watched as they wheeled her down the long corridor and disappeared into the elevator. I turned and looked one last time into the room she vacated. It was empty, dark, and eerily still. All of the nurses were elsewhere, and I found myself alone in the ward. Physically tired and emotionally drained from the morning's events, I walked into an empty waiting room just down the hall and sank into one of the plush lounge chairs. I needed to take a breath and collect my thoughts.

While my mind was still trying to absorb everything that had happened over the last couple of days, denial firmly obstructed it. I couldn't accept the fact that Mom was dying, even with all of the evidence. It was as if I were living in someone else's world, and I was just along for the ride. At any moment, I thought, someone is going to walk up to me and slap me hard in the face. When they do, I'll find myself waking from a hellish nightmare. I'll sit up in bed, rub the sleep from my eyes, and laugh at the absurdity of it all. It will dawn on me that Mom and Dad are home in bed or traveling the world on a cruise ship. I sat there, waiting in the stillness. No one came to wake me up.

As I leaned forward to massage my temples, I noticed some brochures that were scattered about an end table adjacent to where I sat. The topmost pamphlet was titled, "Gone From My Sight: The Dying Experience." I picked it up, read the first few sentences, and began to cry. I wasn't dreaming. It was real. Mom was dying. It was the first time that the reality of it all began to set in.

Sunday, December 4

My sisters spent the first night with Mom and Dad. Glen and I came over early Sunday morning to relieve them and offer any help we could, but most of all just to be there with Mom. We were all happy she was home, and we all wanted to be with her. Mom was weak, but able to talk and carry on a coherent but slurred conversation. Countless times she asked that we would all stop fussing over her.

"Go home," she said. "You don't have to be doing all of this. You need to be with your families."

When we rejected the idea, we received the "evil eye." It was a purposeful glaring look, but it was obvious there were no daggers behind it. It had no impact whatsoever, and she knew it. We just smiled in loving defiance and carried on. I probably would have said the same thing, but none of us was going to leave unless it really upset her.

She was always an independent woman, a matriarch in every sense of the word, who helped others. She worked closely with the church, helping out in any way she could by cleaning and providing funeral lunches for parish families who lost loved ones. Now she was on the receiving end, and the attention was uncomfortable for her.

Mom was going to receive her first visit from a hospice nurse at ten o'clock that morning. We were all anxious to meet her. I wasn't confident we were doing all of the right things, so validation from a trained hospice nurse seemed essential. Questions, even nonsensical ones, raced through my mind. Were we doing the right things? Were we saying the right things? Would the nurse approve or oppose our caregiving approach? Hospice was so foreign to all of us. I felt clumsy and inadequate at it. We were, in essence, learning the language of death.

At one point, Mom asked to rest in her own bed. We delayed the transfer and explained that it would be best if the nurse could see her first. It was difficult to reason with Mom that way. We were now making the decisions for her, and it agitated her. Here we were, reluctantly weighing Mom's wishes against the possible disapproval of a nameless professional, but it felt like the right thing to do. Dad began to pace the living room floor. I leaned forward off the edge of the couch to keep watch through the sheer curtains on the front window. If I could have wished the nurse to show up in the circle drive that minute, I would have. She was already a half hour late. That half hour turned quickly to an hour, then beyond. My sisters and I pestered Dad to call the hospice office. I suppose he didn't want to appear overanxious, but none of us could stand the wait any longer. Dad finally called from a bedroom phone so that Mom could not hear the conversation. He returned to the living room a few minutes later and informed us that someone would call shortly with a status.

Mom asked, again, to move to her familiar bed. Once again, we denied her the wish. Her patience was running thin, and she inquired as to when the nurse would arrive. We could only tell her that it would be soon, when, in fact, we didn't know at all. Another hour passed, and we were all consumed by frustration and anguish. Dad made another call to the company. We could hear his muffled demands from down the hall. When he returned this time, he was visibly upset and nearly in tears.

"The nurse is in South St. Louis County!" His broken voice fluctuated between whispers and choking protest. "She's got several other stops to make and probably won't be here 'til evening."

We were all angered with the revelation. Even if our nurse left immediately from her current location, it would be over an hour before she arrived. And she still had stops to make. How could they do this to us? How could they be so callous? I was livid. The woman who explained hospice care to us and helped us through the registration process had flat out lied. She made promises the company couldn't keep. It seemed the lowest of lows that they could treat dying people with such disregard. Our whispering disdain had unintentionally elevated to such a volume that Mom could sense something was wrong.

"She's not coming, is she?" Mom's voice was soft and waning.

We explained that the nurse was running late. Mom could only muster a disgusted sigh. It was a moment that plunged me into new depths of anger. Mom felt as betrayed by them as we did. Her journey to life's end was nowhere near the intimate, peaceful, and loving separation that was explained to all of us by the seemingly caring hospice enlistment nurse. In fact, it was the opposite. Mom's hospice care hadn't even started yet, and it was turning out to be the most flagrant disregard for human life I had ever experienced. I began to recognize hospice as a business like any other—its purpose, to make money. My mother was not a human being but a commodity of their trade. She was a source of revenue for their business. I felt they were killing my mother faster than the cancer and with little compunction.

It was, I believe, the turning point for all of us. While common sense should have directed our actions, it didn't. We let the accounts of a seemingly uncaring business, and faceless human beings, dictate our behavior. We were lost meandering puppies, at least until now. Half a day had been wasted on worry and anger. It was a half day we'd never get back with our mother. Half a day, gone.

Almost simultaneously, the lot of us turned our attention to where it was needed most—Mom. We asked her if she would still like to be moved to her own bed. She had no doubts in her mind. She wanted out of the uncomfortable stainless steel contraption as soon as possible. With a sibling on each arm, one in front to lead and another in back to monitor, we lifted Mom from the bed and escorted her down the hall. She could barely walk on her own. Her bare feet shuffled across the carpeted floor in a walking motion, but supported very little.

We sat her on the edge of her soft bed, adorned with a floral comforter and plush pillows. Dad lifted her feet and guided them to the center of the bed while my sisters primped over her pillow and pajamas to make her as comfortable as possible. As Dad brought the comforter over her shoulders, Mom let out a long sigh. I think it was the first time she felt at home since she had arrived. After a few minutes, she drifted off to a deep sleep.

With Mom resting comfortably in her familiar bedroom down the hall, it gave us all a chance to talk openly about what had transpired, or not transpired, with the hospice company. The longer we discussed it, more questions were raised than answers. If the nurse had shown up on our doorstep now, we probably would not have let her in. I have never been a proponent of shooting the messenger, but at this point she was the only physical tie between us and the hospice company she worked for. By now, despite not knowing her name or who she was, she was an invisible representative of a failed commitment.

It was then that Dad provided a revelation that had escaped us all. We didn't have to go with this company. We could switch at any time. Before the words had passed over his lips, I was ready to change. So were my sisters and brother. Dad wasn't completely convinced, however. He wanted to give them a chance, and his reasoning, although hard for us to swallow, was fairly sound. None of us had ever experienced hospice before. When it came to hospice care, we were all naive. Maybe, he convinced us, we should first meet the nurse and go from there. If she didn't possess the skill and compassion we had hoped for, and couldn't commit to the schedule that was documented, then he would change providers. He further explained that there were obviously other sick and dying people out there that the hospice nurses were caring for. If it were Mom being attended to, he would want it to be a quality visit, not rushed just because there are others to see before the day ends.

Dad had always been a very forgiving man. It is one of his finest qualities. As much as he made sense, it was difficult for me to rally around his thought process. It was my dying mother who was taking the brunt of all this. As selfish as it was to think, I didn't care about the others out there. I only wanted what was best for Mom, whatever that was. But it was also his dying wife. If that's what he wanted, I would support it.

It was nearly five o'clock in the afternoon and the whereabouts of the visiting nurse was still unknown. We were frustrated and famished. Lunchtime had passed us by without as much as a whisper, so we decided to call out for pizza. We made joking references to the fact that the pizza delivery man was timelier than the hospice nurse. As hungry as we were, we sat around the kitchen table and picked at our slices of pepperoni and sausage. Dad carried his paper plate into the living room where he could keep an eye on the court that sloped downward toward the main subdivision road. Mom and Dad's house was nearly at the end of the subdivision. Few cars drove by, and even fewer drove up into the court where their tan stucco ranch sat quietly at the center.

After checking on Mom, who was still sound asleep, Dad marched into the kitchen to make another call. His patience was gone, and, this time, he did not hesitate about how he felt and what he wanted from them. He demanded that someone, anyone, show up within the hour. After a brief pause in the conversation, it was apparent that the voice on the other end was not accommodating his wishes. He slammed the phone onto the wall-mounted receiver. I had never seen him so angry.

"Dad, I think it's time to switch. They have completely lost all of our confidence and it's only the first day. Any other company has to be better than this," I offered. "I say we switch, and switch now."

My sisters chimed in with the same message. They pleaded with Dad to cut our losses and make a change for Mom's sake. After a brief discussion, we had all reached consensus. Dad immediately put plans into action.

He first called our Aunt Darlene. Her husband, Mom's youngest brother, had passed away from cancer the year before. He asked Darlene about her experience with hospice and inquired as to the company she used. Although the care they provided for her husband was brief—only a few days—she was satisfied with the experience and with the company she had selected. When the conversation was over, Dad shared the news with us. With little deliberation, we were all convinced that this was the company to use. We at least had a reference now.

Our problem was that it was Sunday. Hospice nurses were working, but company offices were closed on Sundays. Any switch, we thought, couldn't be made until tomorrow. We convinced him to call anyway. At least we could get some direction on how to start the process from whoever was on call.

We all gathered around and listened attentively as Dad called the company's after-hours emergency number. As soon as someone answered, Dad began the arduous explanation of the treatment Mom had received from the current provider. He spared no details and left no pause in the one-sided conversation until he knew he had captured the attention of the person on the other end. A silence fell on the room as Dad listened to the caregiver. He answered only with brief "uh huhs." My sisters and brother and I were chomping at the bit to know what was being said, but Dad made no reference or gestures to clue us in.

"Thank you," he finished, "I really appreciate this from you. It means a lot."

Dad hung up the phone. I could sense relief in his tone. "She's coming right over. She can't do anything right now except start the paperwork, but she can arrange it so that the transfer can happen first thing tomorrow morning."

We were all relieved. The woman hadn't even showed up at our door, and we all felt a sense of comfort we hadn't experienced before. Now, it was a matter of meeting her and seeing if she would live up to her commitments. For me it was bittersweet, although bitter certainly prevailed. The whole process of hospice was starting over again. It felt as if an entire year had been torn away from us. With only a limited number of weeks or days remaining for Mom, time was a precious commodity. Tomorrow seemed so far away. I contemplated if the first hospice company realized the true cost of their inaction.

Less than an hour later, the doorbell rang. It was the on-call nurse from the second hospice company. She was true to her word. That alone was enough to satisfy our thirst for any semblance of accountability. When she walked into the living room, she introduced herself as Joan. She conveyed a comfortable and soothing demeanor, the kind of woman whose presence alone brings warmth to a room. We were all greeted with handshakes and hugs, whichever we preferred. She apologized for the lack of compassion by the other hospice company.

Joan also had a familiarity about her. I could have sworn I'd seen or met her before, although I didn't know where that might have been. Perhaps it was her mothering nature and ordinary attire. She wasn't wearing the typical nurse garb. She wore pleated polyester white slacks with a fuzzy earth-tone sweater. It was nothing bright and showy, but nothing plain either. It reminded me of the kind of simple yet refined clothes Mom wore. I accepted her instantly, but with a hint of caution. She hadn't proven herself fully to me, yet.

When the introductions were over, she sat in the center of the living room on a folding metal chair we brought up from the basement the day before. With all of us kids staying at the house now, and the presence of Mom's medical equipment, living room space was at a premium. We circled around her and listened.

Joan had all the answers we were looking for. Rarely did we need to ask a question. Because Mom's equipment was owned by the hospice company, we would have to get a new bed, new walker, new portable commode, new everything. Joan would arrange it so that her company's equipment would be in place prior to the current hospice company retrieving theirs. That way, Mom would not be without a bed or necessary hardware. There would be visitation every day. A nurse would take vitals and assist Mom with any medical needs on Mondays, Wednesdays and Fridays. A caregiver would assist Mom with baths and other personal needs on Tuesdays and Thursdays. If we needed anyone on the weekends, all we'd have to do is call. Unlike the other company, Joan's company had plenty of staff to assist in the immediate area.

Joan also reiterated what our role, and her role, was. It was painful to hear again. There would be no intravenous drips to supplement her diet. If Mom ate and drank on her own, great. If she didn't, it was her body telling her not to, and we were to accept that. Our role was to ease her pain as much as possible and help her with her separation. Nothing would be done by the hospice company to prolong her life. How dreadful it was to hear those words again. We all knew it to be true. We heard the same thing from the last hospice representative. It was all we could do to nod our heads in reluctant agreement.

Joan's gentle and soft-spoken words, detailed and compassionate explanations, combined with her promises to make things happen as quickly and accommodating to Mom as possible, were wonderful music to our ears. Before leaving, Joan gave us all hugs and handshakes again. There were more hugs than handshakes this time.

When the front door closed behind Joan, we all looked at each other and let out a big sigh of relief. It was obvious to all of us we made the right call. If we didn't say once, we said at least a hundred times to each other that evening, "I'm so glad we did that!" If all that was promised was delivered, Mom would get the quality care she deserved.

To respect Mom's privacy, we decided it was best that the girls stay the night again with Dad and help Mom if she needed it. I was to come by tomorrow morning just as I had done today. It seemed to serve Mom best and the schedule suited us all, so I abided by the decision. I kissed Mom while she slept, and left.

Monday, December 5

When I pulled into the driveway, a white cargo van from the new hospice company had already arrived with the equipment. The young men were busy gathering up their belongings as quickly and inconspicuously as they could. I appreciated their respect and quiet diligence. Mom had been moved to her new bed, and the equipment from the previous company lay gathered in the breakfast room ready to be picked up. For me, it served as a reminder of their contempt for human life. The sooner it was disposed of, the better.

I kissed my mother and stroked her forehead. I told her I loved her. She told me she loved me, too. I couldn't get enough of those, and I couldn't stop saying it. Never before had I treasured them as much as I did then. Each one was more special than the last. I welled up inside every time she said it. Her speech had worsened since I'd seen her yesterday, and she appeared weaker. I asked if I could get her anything. She only asked for water. As quickly as I could, I retrieved a glass and filled it with ice and water. I brought the bent straw to her dry, chapped lips. She took only a few sips of the icy refreshment. It was all she could hold and that simple action rendered her breathless.

I went to my sisters, who were gathered in the kitchen, and asked if any of them had lip balm. Sharon knew right where Mom kept it and went to fetch it from the bedroom bath. She stroked Mom's lips with the moistened wax like a mother would a child. I noticed her eyes were scanning Mom's face as she applied the balm. It was the same searching look that I had when I came face to face with Mom. Every blink beckoned the same question, "Why?" I recalled that same painful look from Dad, Laura, Glen, and Diane the evening before. I turned away. Again, my eyes began to pool. It was more than I could bear to see my mother die. It was another to watch the quiet, lonesome agony of my sisters, brother, and father.

"Does that feel better, Mama?" she asked.

"Yes, thank you," she murmured to her caring daughter. "I'd like to go to bed now."

"Do you want to go to your bed?" Sharon asked as she wiped her moistened eyes.

"Yes."

We all sprang into action. Dad darted to the bedroom to pull back the covers and ready the bed for Mom. I lowered the bed rail while my sisters prepared Mom for the journey. It took all of us to carry her. Mom's legs could bear no weight. It was like carrying a fragile rag doll. Her limbs were soft and lifeless. Several times she moaned in pain. All we could do was apologize and keep her moving to quickly end the nauseating motion. The move physically drained her. Like the day before, she drifted off to a deep sleep as soon as her head touched the pillow.

It was obvious we couldn't do this much longer. The movement was becoming almost unbearable for Mom, and we were clumsy at best trying to carry her. Laura, who had been trained in physical therapy in college, came up with an idea. She had a gait belt at home and had almost forgotten about it. It was a simple strap device used by therapists to lift patients from a sitting or lying position. When she returned that evening, she would bring the belt and give us all a course on how to use it. It would make Mom's transfers much easier.

The girls left to get some much needed sleep. Although Mom slept through most of the evening, they had kept a vigilant watch over her through the night. Glen, Dad, and I took the day shift. We frequently checked on Mom who, at one point, was snoring in her deep slumber. It made us laugh. It was a characteristic Dad was all too familiar with, and I had never known. For those few moments, Mom seemed like Mom again.

Dad asked if we would keep an attentive watch while he went to his basement office and caught up on some bills. They had been stacking up on him since Mom fell ill. Ever since they had been married, Mom had always taken care of the checkbook. She even signed Dad's name to his paycheck so many times that Dad was questioned one day by the bank when he provided his own signature. It didn't match the one on file. After some careful screening and a paradoxical explanation, Dad was eventually allowed to deposit his paycheck.

Some of the bills, he was sure, were overdue already, and it wasn't like either of them to be late for a payment. Saving money and having good credit was very important to them, and a characteristic that was instilled in us as long as I could remember. For the next several hours, Dad labored over the bills downstairs while Glen and I caught up on each other's lives.

Around noon, Mom began to stir. I went in to check on her and found her awake and staring out the white-laced curtains on the bedroom window. I sat on the edge of the bed beside her.

"What are you thinking about?" My question was wrought with fear, but it came out anyway. I wasn't sure I wanted to know, or if she wanted to share it.

"Oh, nothing." She turned to me and smiled.

She wasn't a good liar, but I didn't pursue it any further. In actuality, I did want to know. I wanted to know everything she was thinking and feeling. Would it be inappropriate to ask? Was I doing right by her? Was she in pain? Did she have any regrets? Did I ever do anything to upset her? Is there anything she wants me to do for her? Is there anything she wants to do before …?

Question upon question, thought upon thought, flowed through me, and yet fear dammed them all into a muddled pool of madness. For some brainless reason, I permitted none of them to flow past my subconscious. Instead, I turned to what I was most comfortable with, what I cherished most. It was those precious words I longed to say and hear.

"I love you, Mom." After a long warm embrace, I gathered my senses. "Would you like anything to eat? Maybe some soup or something?"

"Sure," she answered. Her eyes turned back to the sun-soaked picture window.

I left the room burying my residual tears into my shirt sleeve to regain composure. As I perused the lower cabinets for a pot, Dad came marching up the steps.

"She wants some soup."

"Really? That's great!" Dad immediately went to see her. I prepared some lukewarm chicken noodle soup, poured it into a covered cup, and brought it to her. Dad took the cup and began to spoonfeed Mom the thin broth with soft noodles. It was an intimate moment for the two of them, looking into each other's eyes as Dad cared for his wife. I left, closing the door behind me, to give them the privacy they deserved.

Several moments later, Dad emerged from the room. He tilted the cup toward me to show what she had consumed. An entangled pile of noodles lay at the bottom.

"She took the broth, but she only ate a few bites of noodles."

It was a good sign. Other than water and canned health drinks, it was the first time since returning home that she had eaten anything solid. If you can call soup solid, that is.

"I want to show you something." Dad's face was stern and his lips tight. He went to his office downstairs and returned with their checkbook in hand. "Look at this," he said. His voice crackled from the onset of another cry. I wasn't sure why he gave me his checkbook. I looked at him for an answer. "Look at the first page. Then look at the last page."

I scanned the first several pages of entries and then flipped toward the end of the ledger. At first, I checked the balance from then and now thinking that this was a financial issue he was trying to convey to me. Then it hit me. My heart sank. I folded it back to the first page and flipped slowly through the ledger.

Mom's cursive handwriting was easily recognizable. She wrote with an artistic style that was all her own. Six months ago, when the ledger entries began, her handwriting was just that—artistic and neat. The latest entries, however, were completely opposite. They were sloppy and uncontrolled—almost as if a third grader had attempted cursive writing for the first time. While flipping page after page of the checkbook, I could see her handwriting deteriorate. The shocked expression on my face said it all. Dad began to break down.

"It was right there, and I didn't even see it."

He was right. But who would have known since Mom carried the checkbook in her purse all of her life? Surely she would have recognized the decline, wouldn't she? Some of the later entries were so bad they were unrecognizable. Even the calculations were off, and there was a solar calculator built into the feminine checkbook cover. But she never said a word to anyone. Did she intentionally hide it from all of us, or was the progression of cancer so slow that she didn't notice the decline herself? Knowing Mom, I believed it to be the former.

The checkbook was just another reminder that Mom was really dying. The small hopes that crept inside me always seemed to swell to unrealistic proportions, such as her desire to eat soup. It was such a positive boost that I began to think, perhaps, Mom had a chance to survive. It felt like some physical phenomenon might delay, if not abort, her death. Those little encouraging signs caused me to negate everything that was taught to me by the doctors, hospice nurses, and pamphlets. Then something like the checkbook came along and steered me back to grim reality.

Hope is often the engine behind a rollercoaster of emotions. It keeps driving us uncontrollably forward to some unknown destiny. One thing we're always taught is to never lose hope. It's the possibility that things might improve, that there could be movement in a positive direction. The problem with hospice care is that those little upward blips are fleeting and often followed by a steep decline. We're just along for the unsettled, and often demoralizing, ride.

Later that evening, Laura, Sharon, and Diane returned for the night shift. Before I left, Laura provided us all instruction on how to use the gait belt. She demonstrated it with Diane first. It looked simple enough. All we had to do was strap it around each other's waist, grasp it with both hands, and lift with our legs. After the lesson, we practiced on one another. It was a comedy of errors. We tripped all over the place and fell down like children trying to lift each other from a kitchen chair. Mom would be in serious jeopardy if any of us, other than Laura, had to use the contraption. The idea was sound. All we needed was practice, Laura, and a little luck.

Tuesday, December 6

When I returned in the morning, I noticed Mom was back in her hospice bed. Dad and the girls were slouched on the living room furniture. Exhaustion consumed them. It had been a bad night for everyone.

Late that evening, Mom had soiled herself in bed. It took all of them a good portion of the night to clean her, dress her, and move her back to the hospice bed. Mom was so frail, and her skin so sensitive, that the gait belt was of little use. With all of the excessive tugging and pulling, it seemed to do more harm than good.

Mom began to stir, so I went to her. I smiled and hugged her. She looked at me for a moment, then said something I will never forget.

"I don't think God wants me." Her voice was broken and frail. She followed her revelation with a subtle smile that projected a hint of disgust. It hit me like a brick. Here was a God-fearing, devoted, Catholic woman who felt God was turning his back on her.

"How can you say that, Mom?" I beseeched, sitting down beside her.

"I keep asking him to take me and he won't do it. I don't think he wants me."

We gathered around her. We were all deeply affected by the almost injurious comment.

"Don't say that, Mom," Laura insisted.

"Maybe we're praying to keep you around a little more. Did you ever think of that?" My voice broke and a rain of tears began to fall on us all.

"We want you here with us," Laura continued. "God can wait a little while, can't he?"

"Besides," I, once again, turned to the only medium I was comfortable with, "I'm sure he knows he'll have his hands full. He needs more time to prepare for you."

It brought a smile, but it was obvious by the pained look on her face she was ready to go. Cancer had reduced her to a breathing shell of a woman. I thought of the night before when the girls had to cleanse and dress their mother. Mom had gone through the same ordeal with her mother. For a brief period of time, Mom and her sisters took turns caring for their aging mother just prior to placing her in a nursing home. Several times Mom had to clean up after the helpless woman had soiled herself. Years after her mother had passed, Mom made several references that she wouldn't wish that on any of us.

"If I ever get to that point, just put me in a home or shoot me," she'd say.

She said it jokingly, but we knew there was some seriousness to her request. I couldn't help but wonder if the humiliation from last night's episode was the final straw for her.

We were constantly reminded by the hospice staff and doctors that Mom was in no pain. It was difficult to believe considering the visible destruction cancer was inflicting upon her. How would they know, I wondered? How could anyone know, unless they had experienced it firsthand? Perhaps there really was pain that fed her desire to meet God sooner than we desired.

"Are you in any pain, Mom?" I asked.

She shook her head to the contrary in an almost nonchalant fashion, and I could sense it was an honest reply. Thank God, I thought. Thank God.

Just then someone knocked at the front door, opened it, and bid a warm greeting. It was Joan. We were all glad to see her. Her presence alone brought confidence and strength to all of us, even Mom. She went immediately to our mother and tended to her. Dad explained their ordeal the previous night and asked if moving Mom from room to room should be continued. We wanted to grant Mom her every wish, but we were in fear of hurting her even more. Joan agreed that keeping her in the hospice bed was best for everybody.

Then she bent in close and whispered, "Would you like a catheter, hon?"

Mom nodded in approval.

"I've got one in the car," she explained while stroking Mom's face. "I'll get it for you, okay?"

When Joan returned, we provided them privacy by walking out to the cedar deck at the back of the house. It gave some of us the opportunity to smoke. I had quit smoking nearly a year ago, but the urge returned with a vengeance. Diane handed a cigarette to me and one to Dad. Glen and Sharon lit up cigarettes they had brought outside. Laura was the only one who had no vice, no foolish crutch to lean on. We said nothing. We filled our lungs with the blue poison as if it were medicinal and milled about the deck.

Dad, who had never quite given up the habit completely, smoked only when he was out of town on business or playing golf or horseshoes with his Knights of Columbus comrades. He always hid them from Mom. I wondered how he did it so successfully when, as a teenager, Mom knew right off that I had been smoking. She could smell it a mile away. I tried to persuade her it was from the smoky grill at the steak house where I worked after school. She knew better. But how Dad got away with it, I'd never know.

Some of the most absurd thoughts came to mind. As we gathered in silence on the newly built cedar deck, each of us in our own faraway land, I noticed the new stain that had been applied to the wood. Mom was very particular about her things and became distraught when the original stain peeled away from the grain after less than a year. The husband of a friend of mine at work had started a side business stripping and staining decks and fences. I had recommended him to her. I had never met him but had heard from his wife he did good work, was friendly to everyone, and could gossip as well as any woman. He and Mom hit it off. She told me many times what a wonderful person he was and how great a job he did on the deck. Mom couldn't stop talking about him. She even tried to get him to do other chores around the house, which she felt Dad was lagging behind. He would have done them, too, had his wife not reminded him of the insurance risks of doing anything other than deck work.

As I surveyed the deck, I could picture the two of them talking and cutting up. As odd as it may seem, I felt the deck held a special connection among me, Mom, and her handyman. I had brought them together. He had made her happy. Indirectly, I made Mom happy. I wondered if my brothers and sisters had any special connections like that. I'm sure they did, but I never asked openly about it for fear of sounding ridiculous.

I also thought about how senseless it was that most of us were smoking. One would think that going through an ordeal as we were, we would be more mindful of the dangers of smoking. Instead, we turned to them like they were the remedy for our pain. Mom hadn't smoked in over thirty years, yet she was the one with cancer. It just added to the unfairness of it all.

A few minutes later, Joan motioned us through the glass door to return. Dad went immediately to the kitchen sink to scrub the cigarette smell from his hands and face. My sisters and I went to Mom.

"Is Dad trying to get that smell of cigarettes off of him?" she asked with a smile.

In unison we all replied, "You know?" Dad heard the revelation from the kitchen despite his hearing aids being turned down. Mom had always accused him of selective hearing and that moment seemed to validate it.

"Of course," she admitted.

Dad walked in with a kitchen towel cupped in his hands and with surprise emblazoned on his moistened face.

"You knew all along?"

Mom looked at him like a mother would a guilt-stricken child and nodded. Dad embraced her and started to laugh. Mom smiled in the midst of her husband's hug, looked at us gathered around and waved her hand in the air pretending to thwart off the undesirable smell of cigarettes. She made us laugh, unbeknown to Dad who apologized profusely.

"You can't hide things like that from a woman," Joan added with a wink, "We always know."

Joan patiently waited for the couple to part and then began her routine. She checked Mom's blood pressure and vitals, noting the details on her clipboard.

"Is there anything you need?"

Mom's lips muttered, "No," but no sound came from her.

Joan turned to us and reiterated her point of keeping Mom in the living room bed. "I think it's best if she stays in this bed. Moving her between rooms is probably getting very painful for her, and I'd hate to see her get hurt." Joan turned to Mom who was watching and listening intently. "Don't you agree?"

Mom nodded her head ever so slightly in approval, but I could tell it disappointed her.

"I know you miss your bed, Elaine, but your family is taking good care of you and you need to rely on them. You've taken care of them for so long, right?" Joan and Mom smiled at each other. I could sense an understanding in their exchange, like a bond only mothers could share. "Now, it's your turn. Let them take care of you."

The lot of us gathered around the bed and responded nearly in unison, "Yeah, Mom. Let us take care of you now."

Joan gathered her medical instruments and prepared to leave. "Be sure to call me if you need anything, okay?" Before parting she bestowed warm hugs to all of us. With each visit we all felt closer to her. By now, Joan was one of the family. She had earned our trust by living up to her word and supporting our family with a personal and nurturing touch. We would have done anything for her.

Moments after Joan departed, there came another knock at the door. The front entrance, which stood silent for most of the latter part of its existence once we were all grown and moved away, seemed to come to life again the last few days as a revolving door, bringing visitors, caregivers, and well-wishers.

This time, it was my Aunt Darlene. Her husband, Don, the second youngest in a family of eight siblings of which my mother was the baby, had died of cancer the previous year. Darlene had always been a warm and caring woman, the type that brought solace to anyone around her. She possessed a cunning sense of humor and an infectious laugh, although somewhat muted since the recent loss of her husband. Don and Darlene had been wonderful dancers. It was dizzying just to watch them spin and twirl on the dance floor. My wife, an energetic dancer in her own right, asked Don to dance during the wedding reception of his daughter. It was the only time I had seen my wife so winded that she had to sit down and catch her breath.

After an exchange of warm embraces, Darlene pulled a kitchen chair up to Mom's bedside, bent over her, and took Mom's hand in hers. In a quiet whisper, Darlene began to speak. Mom listened intently as they gazed into each other's eyes. I couldn't hear what Darlene was saying, but whatever it was, it held Mom captive. It was a moment where souls are conjoined, where two people unite in body, mind, and spirit. I was awestruck by the tranquil, but intense, energy that connected them. Darlene leaned back and gave a reassuring smile. Mom smiled back, all the while still looking into Darlene's comforting eyes.

"Would you like Communion, Elaine?" Darlene asked.

Mom nodded with approval. Darlene, now a deaconess of her parish, reached into her purse and extracted a pocket-sized Bible and a small brass cylinder that safely cased the blessed wafers of bread. She flipped the red ribbon protruding from the pages of her tiny Bible and began to read. We bowed our heads and prayed with her. With clasped hands and an expression of serious determination, Mom closed her eyes tightly and mouthed the familiar words. When the prayer ended, Darlene unhinged the brass container and pulled a host from it.

"Body of Christ."

"Amen." Mom's response was weakened, but she stressed it with as much devotion as she could muster. Darlene placed the host on Mom's extended tongue. She must have noticed the dry mouth and chapped lips.

"Would you like some water? Would that help?"

Mom declined. Being the purist she was, washing down Holy Communion with water would be sacrilegious, and she would have none of it. Mom clamped onto the wafer with clenched dry lips and slowly absorbed it into her soul.

For the next hour or so, Darlene stayed vigilant over Mom, caressing her arms and holding her hand. There were moments of silence in which they just looked at each other. They were tacit moments, where the unspoken words forged an accord and understanding between the two. I was quite sure the reunion was flooding back memories of her husband's final days. As much as I valued the visit, I felt remorse for Darlene who was reliving the experience all over again. It was bittersweet in every sense of the word.

Mom broke one of the silent pauses with a promise to "keep Donny in line up there."

"That will be a fulltime job, Elaine," Darlene retorted. "I couldn't do it when he was alive, so I don't know what makes you think you can."

Mom nodded and winked with confidence that she was up for the task. It made us all laugh. Mom and her brother had been very close. I think she looked forward to seeing him again.

When Darlene left that afternoon, I felt a closeness to her I'd never felt before. She was always a wonderful aunt, but now she was a friend. Darlene understood every emotion, every thought, every feeling we were experiencing. She was fluent in the unfortunate, yet distinctive, language of loss. She was the teacher, and I was her attentive student. I learned more from her that day about the importance of life and the significance of death than at any other time in my life. Her lesson was powerfully delivered, not through books and speech, but with selfless actions and deeds.

When I went home that evening, it dawned on me that last night was the last time Mom would have slept in her own bed. As I snuggled into my bed that night, I tried to imagine myself in her place. I loved my bed, despite the lumps and sags I continually complained about. It's a warm, safe, comforting feeling being tucked away in your familiar bed, in your familiar room with its familiar shadows and distinct sounds, and with your familiar partner. Mom would experience that no more. It was yet another freedom taken away from her during her arduous journey to death that we all seem to thoughtlessly underappreciate, if not completely disregard.

I laid awake for hours thinking about everything that had transpired, from Mom's distressing revelation of God's denial into heaven, to Joan's and Darlene's visits. Mom may have thought that God didn't want her, but the fact of the matter was, I was not yet ready to give her up. It seemed selfish. It seemed as though I was in a proverbial tug-of-war with God, but I wasn't about to let go. I couldn't.

We were lucky to have Joan and supportive family members like Darlene. I couldn't have wished for better people to help us care for our mother. What a blessing it was to have them, and it was gratifying to me that Mom was getting the best care and support possible.

Wednesday, December 7

I approached the house saddled with trepidation. Opening the front door the last couple of mornings had brought unwelcome changes in Mom's condition. I wondered what would be different today. I paused to prepare myself for what would lie ahead. Besides the unrevealed worsening of Mom's health, Father Ron was scheduled to come over at three o'clock to anoint our mother with a blessing of the sick. It was going to be a difficult and emotional day. I took a deep breath, asked God for strength, and slowly opened the door.

To my surprise, everything looked as it had the day before. Mom was lying on her side and awake. She smiled when I entered the room. I was relieved to see there had been no noticeable decline in her health, and she seemed to be as attentive and mindful as yesterday. I kissed her cheek and bid her a warm greeting.

"How are you feeling today, Mom?"

"Eh, could be better," she wearily replied after taking a deep breath. Then she furnished her trademark grin. Mom still had a sense of humor, although melancholy at best. The more I spoke to her, the more I began to realize there were subtle changes in Mom's condition since last night. Every sentence was broken into segments. It was as if she were blowing up a balloon, taking in a chest full of air between the few words she could muster. Because it was difficult for her to speak, I kept my inquiries to a minimum. She tried to roll over onto her back, but couldn't. She was unable to shift her weight or change positions on her own. Her mobility was confined to limited repositioning of her arms and legs only, and she began to fidget.

"Would you like to lie on your back?"

"Yes, please."

Dad and I carefully rolled Mom onto her back. With Dad on one side and me on the other, we used the fitted bed sheet as an improvised stretcher and moved her body to the center of the bed. The technique was taught to us by Joan as an easy and painless way to shift a bedridden person, and we used it frequently. With the head of the bed slightly elevated most of the time, Mom would find herself slipping down toward the other end. The bed sheet approach was useful to slide her back up into a relaxed position.

After we primped her pillow and bed sheets, Mom motioned to the television. Dad elevated her bed higher so she could see it comfortably while I pulled a series of DVDs from her collection. Dad filtered out the ones he thought she would especially enjoy. They were mostly animated Disney films that she loved to watch. All day she drifted in and out of sleep, catching parts of whatever movie was on at the time, and then slumbered off again.

I wondered if Mom really desired to watch television, or just wanted Dad and me to focus on something else besides her. In either case, it served more as white noise than anything. Dad and I may have been looking toward the direction of the television, but neither of us was really watching it. My peripheral senses, now trained like radar in Mom's direction, were heightened to familiar levels ever since she was delivered home. I could perceive the slightest movements and sounds, even from the next room. It reminded me of a time when my newly born children were first brought home from the hospital. Every unfamiliar sound, or uneasy feeling for that matter, triggered me like Pavlov's dog to stop what I was doing and check on Mom.

I pulled up a chair next to Mom's bed and sat with her for several hours. I kept glancing at her to see how she was doing. Congestion was building in her lungs, which caused her to struggle for each breath. She was getting weaker. During one of the neglected films, she woke up and smiled. I told her I loved her. Her lips mouthed the words I longed to hear, but her words were silent. She turned away and drifted off to sleep again.

At midday, while Mom was still asleep, I went outside to get some fresh air and reflect. It had begun to snow. A thick wet snow came down in large flakes. The deck and yard were covered within minutes. The snowfall brought a peaceful stillness. You could almost hear the flakes touch each other as they crisscrossed the sky and settled into their placid blanket. Missouri didn't see snow like this very often. It was then I prayed to God to take me instead. I offered my life to Him in exchange for hers. She spent most of her adult life raising the six of us. She went to church every weekend and was active in the parish. Her faith was unwavering. There were times we didn't see eye to eye, but she was a wonderful person and didn't deserve to die so young. She was just starting to enjoy her life.

I, on the other hand, was a poor example of a Catholic. In grade school I served Mass often. During the summer, my mother would wake me at five o'clock in the morning every weekday. I gobbled up the freshly cooked oatmeal Mom had prepared, then excitedly rode my bicycle to our small country church to ring the bell and serve the weekday Mass for the few who attended. Somehow, over time, the passion I once felt for attending church diminished. As an adult, I rarely went to Mass. My faith was such that, as ludicrous as it might sound, I believed in God, but I didn't feel the need to go to church to pray. Every time I saw an ocean, or a mountain, or a snowfall for that matter, I had no doubt in my mind He existed. Only God could create something so magnificent. Mom knew of my secular transformation and didn't approve, but she never pressed the issue with me. It just didn't seem fair to take her before me. I prayed He was listening. If He would have shown up that moment to take me up on the offer, I wouldn't be here today.

My mother was also a great believer and avid collector of angels. They could be found in every room of the house, in pictures, statues, plates, and jewelry. Mother's Day often brought more of the collectibles from her children. Two tiny angel statues adorned the steps of the deck. Snow began to collect on the fragile, unclothed beings. Both were beautiful winged creatures, with wavy hair and plump bellies, which were forever cast into a slumped and weeping position. Each had an arm raised to dry the tears from its eye. I often thought they were morbid. Of all the graceful and spiritual poses angels are frequently crafted, why on earth would Mom choose those that are weeping? Several times I had questioned her on her choice. She only responded that she liked them. After all, they were completely opposite of her demeanor.

Mom was an outgoing person, always positive in thoughts and action. If any one of us ever needed to find her at a party or outing, all we had to do was look for a group of people. She could always be found in the center, carrying on and keeping the others in stitches. She also knew how to stand her ground. I suppose it was the stern German upbringing that made her that way. It was a rare occasion for anyone to win an argument with her.

Despite her sometimes stubborn disposition and through the entire plight of her illness, I never once doubted that angels were watching over her. The times I went outside to regain my composure, I stared at the saddened angels. They were now representative of something real. It was as if they mourned for my mother. As much as I despised the poignant creatures before, I was now appreciative of their empathy. Her little guardian angels were there for her.

By three o'clock, our family was gathered together in preparation for the parish priest's visit. Father Ron was due at any time to administer the healing sacrament, the Anointing of the

Sick. I remembered all too well from my grade school religion classes what name it used to be referenced. In my days of Catholic learning, it was presented as the seventh sacrament and the final one to be administered. As one of the Last Rites, it was the Final Anointing, or Extreme Unction, dispensed only to those in immediate peril of death. It was the final provision of faith for the journey of the dying. Its new name, as well as its relaxed usage to those beyond mortal danger, did little to ease my mind.

Unlike baptism and matrimony, which were joyous occasions for celebration, Mom was going to receive what I considered to be the dreaded sacrament. I felt a sense of uneasiness that left me fidgety and agitated. I paced the floor and wandered about the house like a lost visitor. The curtains to Mom's life were gradually being drawn closed. It was an anxious and surreal time waiting for the priest to arrive.

Father Ron arrived right on time. He tapped his shoes on the porch step to rid them of the freshly packed snow and walked in. He was a soft-spoken elderly man of the cloth with salt-and-pepper hair and an honest and gentle demeanor. His words of condolence, as he met with each of us, were genuine and comforting. Of all the parish priests, he was Mom's favorite, and I could instantly see why. He seemed to understand our plight, and his presence alone eased our anguish. He went to Mom and placed his hand on her forehead.

"God is with you, Elaine. We're all praying for you." Father Ron wasted no time. He motioned for us to gather around him and he went right to work.

"Let us pray." He removed a Bible from his trouser pocket and began to read the prayers for the sick.

We bowed our heads and prayed with him. Every phrase, every mention of death, heaven, and life ever after sent a stabbing pain to my heart. The familiar quotations from his tiny booklet were more dreaded affirmations that Mom would not be with us much longer.

During each prayer, Mom looked into his eyes and listened intently to every word, acknowledging each reading with a solemn, "Amen."

The priest then closed the book and pulled a brass vessel from the breast pocket of his black jacket. It was the same kind Darlene carried with her. As he opened the lid, the fragrance of his holy oil wafted in the room. It was a sweet scent, like that of a fresh spring rose garden covered in early morning dew, that brought a spiritual peace to the darkened room. With a dip of his thumb, he lifted a trickle of the aromatic oil and swabbed the sign of the cross on her forehead and chest.

"In the name of the Father, the Son, and the Holy Spirit. Amen." Father Ron then bent over his worthy parishioner, closed his eyes and whispered a private prayer. He seemed to pour out his soul in a divine council reserved only for Mom and him. It was as if he were providing a celestial conduit to God. It was spiritually moving and brought tears to us all.

When he finished his supplication, Father stood erect and turned to us with a smile. The sacrament had been delivered. The ritual concluded. Mom now had the necessary prerequisite for the afterlife.

Father Ron picked up his belongings, slid them back into his jacket pocket and bid farewell. He noted to each of us that it wasn't up to us what happened next. It was all in God's caring hands. In parting, he instilled in us that she was lucky to have such a large and loving family. As logical as it probably should have been to us all, it was a much needed endorsement to hear his words of praise and encouragement. We fell silent as the door closed behind him.

I was trying to grasp everything that had happened. It was an experience that left me in a confused state of dejection and contentment. I was happy for Mom. She was readied for her passing. But the time was drawing nearer, and now we had to resentfully prepare ourselves for that awful moment when God took her from us.

Joan showed up at our doorstep just as the priest was driving away. She must have seen him. It was either that, or the look of despair in our faces that she witnessed upon entering the room. We didn't greet her with hugs and well wishes this time. Instead, we acknowledged her with smiles and somber hellos without moving from where we stood or sat. We didn't intend to be rude, and I hoped it wouldn't be construed as such. We were all still grappling with the significance of the priest's visit.

Without questioning our observable change in disposition, Joan walked quietly to Mom and began her routine examination. While tending to Mom's vital signs, Joan's cell phone rang. She excused herself and walked into the kitchen to take the call. It was obvious from the bits and pieces of her discussion that someone had recently died. She whispered instructions to the caller on how to handle the arrangements. I was relieved that Mom was incapable of hearing the conversation. As demoralizing as it was for us to hear, I couldn't imagine how Mom would have felt had she heard any part of it.

It was a harsh awakening. Soon, although we didn't know how soon it would actually be, Joan would have the same conversation with us. None of us uttered a word. We stood quietly in the living room trying not to let Joan, or each other, know we were eavesdropping.

When she returned, she seemed distraught. The conversation appeared to have struck a personal chord. If she took every death as personally as this one, I thought, what a miserable job to have. How could a person go day in and day out being affected by death in such an intimate way?

When Joan returned to the living room, Dad was the only one to acknowledge her unconvincingly suppressed anguish.

"Are you alright?" Dad, despite his own suffering, was openly concerned for Joan.

"Yes. It was about my mother. She passed away Sunday, and I'm trying to make the arrangements for her."

Our hearts fell with a heavy thud to the floor. We were all in shock. I was mortified. I felt guilty for the burden we had bestowed on this poor woman. Here we were, putting the full weight of our mother's care on the shoulders of a woman who had just lost her own mother. All this time, she had never said a word. We poured out our heartfelt condolences and hugged her like she was our own mother.

Joan reached into her purse for a tissue to dry her eyes. "It's okay," she insisted. "She had been ill for quite some time, so it wasn't unexpected. I'm the only child, and I'm trying to make all of her arrangements."

We apologized profusely and encouraged her to go, but Joan would hear none of it.

"I need to be here for your mother." She returned to Mom to finish her examination. "There's nothing I can do now for mine. I'm happy knowing she's in a wonderful place."

Mom peered into Joan's eyes as Joan concentrated on the echoed sounds emanating from her stethoscope. She must have noticed the stare from Mom and looked at her.

"I'm so sorry," Mom wheezed to her troubled caregiver.

Joan was taken off guard by the consolation from her dying patient. She stroked Mom's face and smiled, all the while fighting back her emotions. A silence blanketed the room. Mom's words left all of us speechless. It shouldn't have surprised us that Mom would do that. It was her nature. But to think of someone else even while she was dying was unimaginable. Mom was a wonderful and giving person, even near the end of her own life.

Joan, being the consummate caregiver she was, gathered her senses along with her tote bag. "I want you to concentrate on your mother. She needs you."

One by one we embraced her like family. None of us let her leave without conveying that she was in our thoughts and prayers. Although we knew Joan would never take us up on our proposals for assistance, we offered anything and everything to her if she needed it. She was grateful for our submissions, but never accepted them. She said good-bye and left.

For the next hour or so, while Mom slept peacefully from her arduous day, we talked about Joan. She had profoundly impacted us all. It was, to say the least, a double-edged sword. Joan was a rare individual, and we were lucky to have her, but how heart-crushing to have her under such dreadful circumstances. In our minds, she was nothing short of a saint.

The events of the day left us exhausted. We each milled about the house in a silent shell, taking care of dishes, bathrooms, or unmade beds. We did not speak to each other. I think we all needed time to digest the day. I know I did.

After a long period of individual isolation, our attention returned to Mom. It started when Laura pulled a booklet from her purse. I recognized it as the same booklet I picked up from the waiting room when Mom was transported from the hospital—"Gone From My Sight: The Dying Experience" by Barbara Karnes.

"Did you see how Joan checked Mom's legs?" None of us had noticed it. "I was reading this book last night, and I think we all need to read it. It talks about the different stages of dying and points out the things we need to look for. Joan was checking her legs for mottling. I hate to say this, but Mom is showing symptoms described in this book, and I think she is very close."

Together we raised the blanket to survey Mom's legs. They were pale yellow with purplish blotches from her knees to her feet. Her hands showed the same discoloration. Circulation to her outer extremities was already starting to fail. Laura's revelation was yet another awakening for all of us. There was no turning back. Mom's death was drawing closer.

Throughout the evening, we each read the booklet. It was only fourteen pages long, but it packed more insight into what Mom was experiencing than any of us could possibly imagine. As each of us finished the book, we fell into a melancholy state of mind. We said nothing to each other. What else was there to say? The book said it all. It explained what we could expect from months, to weeks, to days, to hours, to the final minute of death. Mom was showing all of the signs of being within one week to just days from separation. Her skin was translucent and clammy. Her breathing was congested and labored. She drifted off to sleep more often while her eyes were only half open. The book was prophesizing everything, even to the most negligible detail.

Being newly adept in the physical signs of dying, we all had a better understanding of the changes Mom was going through and how much time we had with her. That evening we each held her, touched her, and spoke our most genuine thoughts. Whether she could hear us or not, we wanted her to know how much we loved her.

Thursday, December 8

I was sound asleep when the phone rang. It startled Patti and me. From the pit of my conscience I heard someone mutter, "Oh, no." It was my voice, but it never escaped my lips. I cursed at the thought of Mom passing away while I was at home in bed and that my family was alone struggling with the pain. I squinted at the brash red numbers on the alarm clock until they came into partial focus. It was just before midnight.

"Hello," I sleepily answered. It was Laura.

"Mom is moaning and gasping, and she's not responsive," she said with a nervous tone. "We've called the hospice nurse. It's really bad. We don't know what to do."

"Do you think it will be tonight?" I asked.

"I think so. It's really bad, Doug."

I paused for a minute trying to bring some focused thought on the somber subject. "When will the nurse be there?"

"We left a message. We're waiting on her to call us back."

"Well," I couldn't gather an ounce of sensibility, "do you want me to come over?"

"I don't know," Laura sighed. Her thoughts seemed as muddled as mine.

"Call me after you talk with the nurse, okay?" She agreed and we parted with the briefest of good-byes. I lay in bed for several minutes trying to gather my senses.

I had had second thoughts about leaving Mom that evening, but Dad convinced me to go and promised he would call if there were any changes. I should have stayed, I thought to myself. I should have stayed.

"What's the matter?" Patti asked.

"It's Mom. She's not doing well. They think it might happen tonight." My eyes started to adjust to the faint light from the moonlit bedroom windows and our daughter's night light from down the hall. Blurred shadows of picture frames and furniture began to gain focus. At that moment, thoughts turned to action, and I shot out of bed.

"I need to go over there."

My clothes from last evening were crumpled on the floor of the bedroom closet. I gathered my wrinkled jeans and flannel shirt and dressed. To cover my bedraggled hair, I quickly retrieved an old baseball cap from the closet shelf and hurried out of the house.

When I arrived, I noticed a handwritten sign taped to the front door that read, "Please enter through garage." Throughout the week, as people had entered and left through the front door, the temperature in the living room dropped at least ten degrees as the winter winds quickly swirled through the house. We were always cognizant of the draft and quickly shut the door behind us. Dad, I thought, must have grown tired of securing the entryway and put up the sign to protect Mom, especially now that she was in such a fragile state. I ran around the front of the house and through the opened garage. Upon entering the kitchen, I could hear Joan talking with the family. I thought I was too late.

As I rounded the corner from the kitchen to the living room, I could see Joan caressing my mother's arm and talking in her usual gentle and calming way to my father, brother, and sisters, who were gathered around the bed. She had a natural comforting way about her, but this time, it seemed more apologetic. My first thought was that Joan was consoling them. Dad's expression was that of shock. His hand was wrapped tightly around his mouth.

"No," I thought to myself, "Please, no." A rush of emotions came over me and left me so flushed, it completely took away the winter chill from my body. I was angry with myself, sad, and hurt all at the same time. My knees wobbled and my heart pounded against my chest. The sensation swallowed me so fast I wanted to collapse. It was imperative that I be with her when she passed, but for some senseless reason, I didn't think it would be tonight. I thought I had a little more time. Was this going to be yet another regret piled onto the heap of regrets that already burdened me? I wanted to kick myself for being such a selfish fool.

Then I heard Mom gasp. I wasn't too late, but what I saw at that moment would haunt me forever. Mom's eyes were open wide and her jaw appeared unhinged as she stared into the nothingness in front of her. A black film had formed in the white of her eyes, starting from the outer most points and spreading inward toward her soft auburn pupils. It reminded me of the awful cancer that had brought her to this state. It was deeply disturbing to see, and I wondered if Mom was still gifted with sight. The expression on her face was that of terror. It was as if she had just rounded a corner and found herself standing face-to-face with a horrific monster—motionless and stunned.

Every breath came in slow intervals. Each one was labored and appeared painful. As she exhaled, her lungs gurgled with liquid. A sound like that of a pot of boiling water emanated from her chest long after all of the air had been expelled. Then came the long silence. It was during those seconds of stillness, although it seemed like an eternity, that I wondered if the previous breath was her last. As much as I wanted my mother to be with us, part of me wanted it to end. No living thing should be put through such torment. The momentary restful silence was soon broken by another ghastly inhale. It was as if a sword had been thrust into her heart. Mom's back arched with every intake of precious air, and each wail crushed our souls. Being unaccustomed to Mom's latest condition, I began to count the seconds between breaths. They were anywhere between five and seven seconds apart. It seemed as if she were going to die at any moment. I was crushed at the sudden turn of events. My soul screamed for it to stop.

Joan must have seen the disbelief etched on my face. She tried to explain that, despite how it appeared, it was normal. Perhaps to take our minds off the horrific scene, Joan began to enlighten us on the technical aspects of Mom's condition. She explained that saline drips were not used since they would only draw more water into the lungs. She also insisted that Mom was in no pain, although that was hard to come to terms with given the unspeakable new circumstances. The medical affirmations didn't ease my mind. Everything she said just breezed past me. The uncontrollable gasps brought tears to my eyes. As I bent over my mother to hug her, my tears moistened her cheek. She offered no indication that she knew I was there. For me it was another tragic awakening. Any shred of hope turned to an abyss of despair. Mom was near death, and I couldn't do a thing about it.

"I know," Joan comforted, "I think she is still aware and can hear us, so let her know that you love her."

In just a few hours, Mom's health had declined tenfold. It was then I realized something. I had been given my last hug and "I love you" from my mother. I would never hear those words from her again. I would never feel her arms around me again. Others weren't so lucky, I knew. Few are offered the chance to say their good-byes so many times. But it was heart-wrenching nonetheless. I cherished each one and made the foolish assumption I would be bestowed at least one more. It had only been a few hours, but it seemed like a lifetime ago when she held me. Mom's precious gifts of love would be given no more. It was absolutely devastating. I wanted to die with her.

Joan provided me a small bottle of morphine, although Joan and Mom's doctor had made it clear to all of us that she was not suffering any pain. I think it was more to help ease our pain as we aided our mother in her separation from this life. Joan also placed some glycerin swabs on the bed cart to keep Mom's lips and tongue from drying.

"I would give her several drops of the morphine every two hours, if you feel she needs it. Use the glycerin swabs every hour or so. Just try to keep her as comfortable as you can." Joan buttoned her coat and raised the collar around her neck. It was bitterly cold outside. "If you need anything, or if anything changes, let me know. Okay?" With a warm smile and hugs for everyone, Joan left us.

For the next couple of hours, although it seemed an eternity, the congested inhale and gurgling exhales continued. Dad cried. He prayed that God would just take her now and stop the cruelty. It was the first time I had prayed for the same thing. It's hard to ask God to take someone from you who you love so much. But no one should have to go through what she was going through. No one.

I stayed beside her the rest of the night and into the morning. Glen, Laura, Sharon, and Diane stayed up all night as well. Mom's gasps turned to deeper quieter breaths as time passed and the blank wide-open stare faded to closed eyes. Every hour on the hour, I faithfully moistened her lips with the pungent glycerin swabs. Several times, as the tip of the swab entered her mouth to relieve her dry white tongue, she clamped down so tight I couldn't extract it. All I could do was wait for her jaws to loosen their grip on the medicinal swab, then slowly remove it, careful not to touch her lips for fear she would clamp down on it again. It reminded me of the game of Operation, where young wannabe doctors extract oddly shaped parts from a patient's limbs and torso without setting off lights and buzzers. It made me smile. It was a natural reaction from Mom, her only natural reaction other than breathing that took the emptiness of certain death away, even for just a moment. Every other hour I squeezed a couple drops of morphine onto her tongue. I never knew if she needed it or not, but I wasn't about to take that chance.

Dad had been up for nearly thirty-six hours straight, and he was feeling delirious. We convinced him to go to bed, but only after a solemn promise we would wake him if anything changed. It was up to me and my unflagging younger sisters and brother to keep our vigilant watch over Mom. Laura and Diane took turns napping on the couch or on Dad's plush rocking chair. Sharon slept in the spare bedroom for a few hours and then came back out to join us. Glen caught a few winks on a spare couch in the basement.

I couldn't sleep, although I did drift off on several occasions. I felt compelled to keep the glycerin and morphine schedule. As she slept, we all had become accustomed to Mom's breathing pattern. It was like the steady tick of a clock, or the rhythmic waves of the ocean as they reach for the shore, or the blinking red light of a radio tower. If we sensed any change to the interval, we knew it immediately.

Many times the distance between breaths was more than ten seconds, twice the norm. It was on those occasions we were arrested, waiting for the next breath and ready to spring down the hall to wake Dad if it didn't come. Those who were sneaking winks of sleep, opened their eyes. At one point, Sharon called my name and looked at me with searching eyes. I was already fixated on Mom waiting for the next release of air. Just as we were about to check on her, she exhaled and started the rhythm over again. Our chests deflated as well.

It was the longest night of our lives. We stayed in the dark, quiet living room as Mom's favorite pendulum wall clock swept away time. None of us said a word. We communicated through subtle facial expressions only. Mom's death was drawing closer and we all knew it. It was just a matter of time.

Friday, December 9

As he had done nearly every day since his early retirement, Dad woke from his slumber sharply at four o'clock in the morning and shuffled into the living room. Driving over thirty miles in rush hour traffic all of his adult life had programmed his body to rise early, and it stayed with him long after he retired. It looked as though he hadn't gotten a wink of sleep. He sat next to his beloved wife, stroked her head and began to cry. I updated him on the regular applications of morphine and glycerin and showed him the spreadsheet I had kept throughout the night. It was another one of those inconsequential things that seemed important at the time.

After learning that I had not slept since Wednesday, Dad insisted I go home and get some rest. I rejected the idea at first, but once the seed was planted, it seemed my system began to shutdown. I yawned almost uncontrollably every few minutes as fatigue started to settle in. Just the mention of repose triggered my need for sleep.

Mom hadn't varied from her breathing pattern, aside from several heart-stopping surprises earlier that morning, so I felt comfortable leaving for a few hours to catch up on some much needed sleep. I was in a rare state of exhaustion combined with hyperactive restlessness.

As tired as I was, I knew going to sleep would be nearly impossible. Between digestion of what had transpired until now, and the thoughts of what lay ahead, I had too much to think about to fall asleep. So before I left, I took a pill from one of Mom's prescription bottles—an extra-strength sleeping aid that was prescribed to help her sleep through the nausea that ritually followed her chemotherapy sessions. Living only a few miles away, I washed the pill down with bottled water before I left so that it would kick into gear by the time I arrived home. It did just that. I tiptoed to bed so as not to wake Patti and drifted off to a deep sleep.

The phone rang at eight o'clock that morning. I leaned slowly forward while lying on my back to survey the room. The effects of the sleeping pill were in full force. Patti was gone, presumably at work. I had never heard her leave. There were no muffled sounds of early morning cartoons emanating from downstairs. Paige, our middle-school-aged daughter, must have already left for school. I picked up the phone and disregarded the proper manner of introduction.

"Doug?" came a voice on the other end. It was Diane, I think. It was a woman's voice. That I knew for sure.

"Yeah."

"We think it might be soon."

"Okay, I'll be right over," I muttered to the voice on the other end and hung up the phone. I must have dozed off again. The next thing I knew, Patti was at my side tugging on my shoulder to get up. Diane apparently had attempted to call me earlier that morning, but when I didn't answer, she called Patti at work. As it turned out, it was Patti on the phone. She could tell I wasn't in a rational frame of mind and, considering the grave nature of Diane's call, had left work to get me. I don't remember much from that moment until I arrived at Mom and Dad's house, other than I left a gap in the driver's side window so that the brisk winter air would keep me awake and focused.

Mom and Dad's house. Something about that phrase didn't feel right. Is it Dad's house now? Would it be disrespectful to Mom if we omit her name from the classification that has always been "Mom and Dad's house"? Mom was the one who made the house a home—decorating, furnishing, cooking, cleaning—all the things a good mother and homemaker does. Her refined sense of style could be found in every room of the house, and from floor to ceiling. Crazy were the thoughts that entered my mind on the drive over.

When Patti and I arrived, Heather, the young hospice nurse who came every other day to care for and bathe my mother's weakened body, was leaning over the bed and checking vital signs. The rest of my family was already acquainted with her. It was the first time I had seen Heather since her schedule differed from mine, but I was too delirious for introductions. She wore the typical nurse garb, a colorful flowered smock and white slacks. She quietly sat down at the foot of Mom's bed and wrote notes on her clipboard.

I flopped down on the couch and surveyed the room. Other than Heather's presence, nothing had changed since I had left three hours ago. Mom was still settled into the same restful but labored breathing pattern as when I left. My brother and sisters were scattered about the living room and kitchen and were focused on various tasks around the house. I wondered why I had been called over at all, but I never questioned it aloud. I tried to fight back the effects of the sleeping pill and focus on what was going on. My head bobbed as I drifted in and out of consciousness. Unless I did something quick, I was sure to fall asleep where I sat.

"I'm going to make some coffee," I announced in a mumbled blather as I stood up and walked to the kitchen.

Over the last seven days I had gotten more accustomed to Mom's kitchen than in any other time in my life. I knew precisely where everything was. I felt guilty about it. Why hadn't I known these things before? Why was it that only in death would I come to know my mother's surroundings? Perhaps if I had visited more, or had a deeper relationship while she was healthy, I would have known these things. Even menial tasks as making coffee brought remorse and thoughts of what should have been. Regret after regret paraded through my mind, one after another. I stared into the emptiness in front of me as eight cups of the aromatic liquid dribbled into the carafe.

Before it had a chance to finish brewing, I pulled the decanter from the machine, poured the fresh brew into a large travel mug and laced it with cream and sugar. As I bent toward the sink to rinse the stirring spoon, the morning sunlight streaming through the kitchen window, intensified by the fresh snowfall, struck me square in the face and snapped my eyes closed. I blinked to wash the burned white image from my sight and followed it with several gulps of coffee. The combination of glare and caffeine helped to fight off my pill-induced desire for sleep.

My eyes slowly regained their focus, and the white lustrous landscape of the backyard captured me. I had always referred to it as the "day after" snow, when tree limbs bend to the weight of their pallid companion, and houses and fence rows are adorned like pearl wedding cakes. It was the kind of snow children wished for Christmas—peaceful and pure—ripe for snow angels, forts, and rudimentary carrot-nosed statues. It was truly a beautiful day, despite the circumstance.

Next to the kitchen window hung a gold-framed picture. It bore the words to *Footsteps in the Sand*, by Mary Stevenson. I was familiar with its verse, but felt compelled to read it again.

> One night a man had a dream. He dreamed he was
> walking along the beach with the Lord. Across the
> sky flashed scenes from his life. For each scene, he
> noticed two sets of footprints in the sand: one
> belonging to him, and the other to the Lord. When
> the last scene of his life flashed before him, he
> looked back at the footprints in the sand. He
> noticed that many times along the path of his life
> there was only one set of footprints. He also noticed

that it happened at the very lowest and saddest
times in his life. This really bothered him and he
questioned the Lord about it. "Lord, You said that
once I decided to follow you, You'd walk with me all
the way. But I have noticed that during the most
troublesome times in my life, there is only one set
of footprints. I don't understand why when I needed
you most you would leave me." The Lord replied,
"My son, My precious child, I love you and I would
never leave you. During your times of trial and
suffering, when you see only one set of footprints, it
was then that I Carried You."

I began to cry alone. The burden of my regrets was heavy and
unbearable. It didn't feel as though He was carrying me now. I
thought that my jaded view of organized religion and lack of
religious practice had excluded me from the privilege of being
carried. Perhaps I should learn to bear the brunt of my actions
alone. I wasn't one of the deserved ones like my mother.

As many times as I had hugged my mother and told her I
loved her the past few precious days, it was not enough. I
wanted more. I wanted to say more. I wanted more meaningful
time to spend with her. But it was gone. All gone. I could do
nothing but wait, and think, and wait. It was simply, and horribly, a matter of waiting for Mom to die. None of us would be
gifted hugs, kisses, cards, calls, or laughter from her any more.
Family outings, New Year's parties, Thanksgiving, and Christ-

mas would all be missing a significant ingredient. How on earth could we possibly do any of these things without her? How could we go about our daily life without her? For me, it seemed like the end of the world. Life without Mom was inconceivable. Being alone with one's thoughts can be a dangerous thing. Despite the sun, the fresh fallen snow, and all of my family within arms' reach, it was the darkest and loneliest time in my life.

Just then, I heard Sharon shriek. It broke me from my dispirited musings. Heather beckoned everyone to come to the living room immediately. Then I heard my father cry out. My family circled Mom's bed and began to cry. As I darted around the corner of the bed, I looked at Mom. Mom gasped as though she were startled by something. It was as if she were the recipient of a surprise birthday party where everyone jumped out from hidden corners of the room and yelled "Surprise!" Upon her face was the brightest smile I had ever seen. Her cheeks, pale for days, bloomed like roses. Her lips were alive with color and framed her pearlescent teeth hidden for so long behind a curtain of grimace. It was a smile, a big beautiful smile, genuine in every sense of the word. It was a smile that would live in me forever.

"Is she gone?" someone asked.

"Yes," Heather replied. She also began to well up. "She's gone." Even Heather, a hospice professional for several years, had never seen anything like it.

"Look at that smile," Dad cried out as he cupped his hand over his mouth.

"She's in heaven," Sharon exclaimed.

It was our mother's last respire, but before she left, she gave us a gift of majestic proportions. It was the most honest and naturally beautiful smile I had ever seen. We cried like we never cried before, but our tears were intertwined with happiness. There had been a time when we begged God to take her. The last few days seemed so painful and unfair that we prayed for a quick separation for her sake. I even tried to bargain my life for hers. Our wonderful mother didn't deserve this. Thankfully, our prayers were more than answered. Mom's journey had finally ended, and it ended with a magnificent smile.

Epilogue

My family had known nothing of palliative care prior to our mother's diagnosis of terminal brain cancer. We were thrust into it. It was the proverbial baptism by fire. We might as well have been forced onto a ship and ordered by the captain to sail it to Europe. The task of hospice seemed just as daunting. Like meandering little puppies, we clumsily felt our way through the entire ordeal.

We were lucky to have such a large family to support each other. I couldn't imagine taking on such a responsibility alone. But the term *strength in numbers* didn't seem to apply. We were all equally lost and equally searching for answers.

I think it's impossible to prepare for hospice. One can only experience it. It is the inevitability of it all that is difficult to digest. The only uncertainty is *when*. By its most rudimentary definition, hospice means "accommodation." It was explained to us early on that there would be no attempts to prolong her life or revive or resuscitate from any sudden decline. The function of hospice was to accommodate—to tend to every need of the physical, spiritual, and emotional realms of the sick, without endeavor to heal. It is the final sequel to, "There is nothing more we can do." That is an obstinate pill for anyone to swallow.

Through Mom's entire ordeal, from the moment she was diagnosed with cancer to her miraculous final moment of separation, we never saw her cry. Tears were never shed in front of her children. To this day I'm uncertain whether she held them back as a characteristic of her maternal strength, or if she accepted her fate well before any of her family had.

Like the figurines Mom collected, the experience brought us several "real" angels in Joan and Darlene. Had it not been for their selfless acts of kindness, empathy, and support, the experience would have been much different. We were struggling to provide the best for Mom. We had no confidence that what we were doing was right, despite having consensus in our large family. Joan and Darlene helped not only to validate what we were doing, but to elevate it to a level that was beyond anything we could have imagined. Mom's separation from life was as profound and peaceful as it could have been because of them.

Time was a fickle thing during the entire ordeal. Had it not persisted in its slow methodical march toward Mom's final breath, it would have been considered nearly absent for the rest of us. I can still hear the ticktock of the wall clock in their living room. Other than Mom's labored breathing and periodic whispers from family and visitors, it was the only sound to be heard that entire week. Each swing of its pendulum seemed like hours.

It is amazing to me now how much time we fritter away on nonessential things. Pressures of deadlines and busy schedules were on an unnatural hiatus. Television, radio, newspapers, mail, and Internet correspondence, once important elements of our everyday lives, were loathed distractions. I didn't want to know what was happening around the world. In fact, it is safe to say, I detested any news that reported anything other than the condition of my mother. How could a traffic jam on Interstate 70 during rush hour, or the debate of local city officials over a development project, be of any importance when a woman lay dying in her living room? My perspective has since changed. I find I don't complain about how a snowfall is congesting roadways. Instead, I enjoy the interruption and capture its beauty.

The "awakenings" I referred to were just that. I found it effortless to slip into the warm embrace of hope, time and time again. It's human nature, and without it we find ourselves in a cold heartless place. For two years we declined to believe anything that was contrary to wellness. Like so many other women, Mom had driven breast cancer from her body. If she could do that, she could do anything, including survive her latest afflictions. Through it all, even through the seemingly endless train of bad news, we all held hope that Mom would somehow rise above it all. That was slowly and painfully chiseled away during her last days on earth.

The last seven days of my mother's life were the worst in my family's history. So many times we allowed false hope to bubble up from the churning depths of raw emotion, only to have it burst, expelling noxious fumes in our face. Hope was often our last frontier. How ashamed it was to have it diminished by knowledge and truth, whether from books or medical professionals. But these things, as unwelcome as they were at the time, helped guide our actions and lessened the amount of regret.

Had we not known that our mother's death was as imminent as it was, perhaps we would not have expressed our love as we did.

Once the realization was absorbed that our mother was going to die, hope didn't disappear as I thought it would. Instead, it took on a transformation. Rather than forge desires for a healthy return to life as we know it, we prayed for peace and a painless separation. We asked God to take her tenderly into his arms and make it all the splendor she had faithfully believed for so many years. She held steadfast to her faith in words and action, and she believed that angels were as real as you or I. I hoped that the hereafter would be everything she imagined.

Our hopes were realized in a profound way. What we received was as simple as an honest human reaction, yet it was beyond all comprehension. Hope came in the form of a brimming smile. We couldn't have asked for anything more. To this day I would give anything to see what she saw. Was she welcomed by her deceased family members who were terribly missed on earth? Was Saint Peter waiting for her with open pearly gates? Did a host of angels, similar to the beautiful flowing figurines she collected, deliver her to heaven? Was she happy to know her suffering was over? Will we ever know? Perhaps the mystery is worth the wait.

I miss you, Mother, but I know I will see you again.

978-0-595-46373-2
0-595-46373-8